Healing Oils
of the Bible

David Stewart, Ph.D.

CARE Publications

First printing June 2003 - 2,200 copies
Second printing October 2003 - 3,300 copies
Third printing May 2004 - 5,500 copies
Fourth printing October 2004 - 5,500 copies
Fifth printing August 2005 - 11,000 copies

Publisher's Cataloging–in–Publication
(Provided by Quality Books, Inc.)

Stewart, David, 1937 Sept. 20–
   Healing Oils of the Bible / by David Stewart. -- 1st ed.
   p. cm.
   Includes bibliographical references and index.
   LCCN 2001119975
   ISBN 0-934426-98-8

   1. Bible--Criticism, interpretation, etc.
   2. Essences and essential oils--Therapeutic use.
   I Title.

BS680.05S74 2002   220.8'615321
                                     QBI02-200380

IMPORTANT NOTICE

The information in this book is intended for education purposes only. It is not provided in order to diagnose, prescribe, or treat any disease, illness, or injured condition of the body. The author, publisher, and printer accept no responsibility for such use. Anyone suffering from any disease, illness, or injury should consult with a physician or other appropriate licensed health care professional.

Care Publications

RR 4, Box 646
Marble Hill, MO 63764
(573) 238-4846 or (800) 758-8629
care@raindroptraining.com
www.CarePublications.net
www.RaindropTraining.com

05   06   07   08   09   10   9   8   7   6   5

"This is the best book I have ever read in my life. I finished it in three days despite the fact that I have two young boys (ages 2 and 4). I liked it because it establishes a Biblical basis for the use of essential oils, subjects that I love. I just couldn't put it down and I keep going back."

Kelly Fowler, Homemaker and Mother
Flagstaff, Arizona

"David Stewart has a way of communicating that is easy to read and understand. After reading the book, I immediately ordered another one so that I could share it with others. For me the book brought a union of the physical and spiritual world and helped me to understand that there is much more to healing than just the physical. Dr. Stewart has brought ancient healing practices together with today's science for tomorrow's future."

Nicole Page
Calgary, Alberta, Canada

"This is one of the few books I have ever read that I absolutely could not put down until I finished it. I can't tell you how much I have enjoyed reading this book. It is truly wonderful!"

Owen Newman, Writer and Pioneer Craftsman
Glen Allen, Missouri

"I just received your book, *Healing Oils of the Bible* and am totally fascinated by it. I was up till 4 A.M. reading it! It just amazes me what you have in there. Reading it has been a real awakening for me. I love the way you have it formatted. You can pick any chapter, and it reads as a stand-alone work. As for the Bible Program at the end, I am really touched by your generosity and graciousness. This is a ministry I want to do. I just want to bless you and thank for such a beautiful gift."

Kay Cansler
Asheville, North Carolina

"I just received *Healing Oils of the Bible* a month ago and am now on my third time reading it through. I feel like I have discovered a great treasure chest. I have been a Christian all my life, since earliest childhood, and am discovering things about my faith I never knew before. This book has really opened things up for me. What an exciting book!"

Sherry Reese
Tallahassee, Florida

"This book is magnificent!!! Not often am I moved to not put a book down until it is thoroughly read. Rarely is there a book that I ever read from cover to cover. Your book is an exception. I am fascinated with how such profound truth can be presented with such eloquence and simplicity. Even those without Biblical or traditional church knowledge could read this book and walk away touched by its content. I enjoyed it so much that it even became bedtime reading material to my children. They have enjoyed it almost as much as I have, and that is saying a lot when you consider their ages: 7, 8, and 13. Thank you for letting the truth pour forth from your heart. The passion in how you present this material has profoundly changed me and the lives of my children. I eagerly wait for the second act, but until then I will pray God's bountiful blessings on this breathing masterpiece.

Pati Thayer, CMMT, CNA, CMGC
Paw Paw, Michigan

"In *Healing Oils of the Bible* Dr. David Stewart brings the truth of God,s word into our lives. Dr. Stewart shows us God's desire for us to have lifestyles free of disease. He cites holy scriptures, names specific holy oils, and outlines a Bible Oils Program to encourage us to take responsibility for keeping our bodies sound, vigorous, and healthy. The Bible Oils Program mentions the fragrance of essential oils in the Garden of Eden, teaches the importance of oils in the lives of Biblical people, demonstrates how to use the oils for our benefits today, and concludes with reading James 5:14, calling for the elders of the church to anoint the sick with oil. This must-read book is for every person who desires to know, understand, and use essential oils for improved health."

Rev. Marlene D. Lake, Retired United Methodist Pastor
La Crosse, Wisconsin

"This book cites the Word of God in over 500 scriptures that refer to essential oils and their usage. What a wonderful compilation of factual evidence of the true meaning of healing! David describes the true essence of wellness and documents just how un-natural is the medical view of healing today and the harm we do by using pharmaceuticals. I recommend this book to every medical doctor and urge them to change their paradigm accordingly."

Debbie Allen, CNHP
Denver, Colorado

ACKNOWLEDGMENTS

My wife, Lee Stewart, spent many hours editing and proofing this book and for that I thank her. She made many suggestions that have significantly improved its quality. I also wish to express my gratitude to her for the many things over many months she has done to make it possible for me to write this book. Without her assistance, encouragement, and sacrifice it could not have been done.

There are others whom I also wish to credit for helping create this work. Without the editing, proofing, and thoughtful suggestions of Rev. Jennifer Tilston, of Brevard, North Carolina, Joanne Schwarm, CCI, of Burlington, Iowa, Jacqui Close, CCI, RA, of Jackson, Missouri, Karen Boren, of Payson, Utah, Debbie Allen, CNHP of Denver, Colorado, Mary Ann Hunter of Burlington, Iowa, Kathy Spohn, CCI, of Grand Rapids, Michigan, and Janet McBride of Phoenix, Arizona, this book would have been considerably less than it is.

Cover Art Caption is on the next page . . .

COVER ART

The picture of Mary, Joseph, baby Jesus, and two of the wise men is adapted from a portion of a larger painting by the Italian master, Carlo Dolci (1616-1686). The work is entitled "The Adoration of the Magi." Dolci included a third wise man in his painting just off to the right, not shown in this excerpt. Dolci was one of the most famous artists of his day and painted many religious scenes.

The silver and gold vessels in the center of the picture are incense censers. In Biblical times, hot coals were placed in the bottoms of censers with frankincense, myrrh, onycha, galbanum, balm, and other aromatic gums heaped on a concave metal depression near the top. In the cover picture you can see chunks of the oleo-resins of frankincense and myrrh piled on top of all three censers. When the base was charged with coals, the heat beneath would vaporize the oils whose fragrant fumes would diffuse out of the top or through vents in the lid.

Censers are mentioned 20 times in the Bible. (For example, see Numbers 16:46 or Revelation 8:3-5.)

Dolci's work is on display at the British National Gallery in London who kindly provided a transparency from which this cover was produced. Dolci's painting can be viewed in its entirety on the web at:

<www.NationalGallery.org.uk>

Table of Contents

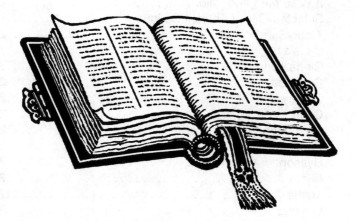

Introduction

Healing Versus The Practice of Medicine

The purpose of this book is to educate and inspire you to realize the infinite care and detail to which our creator has gone to provide for us the medicines we need to heal and maintain our health. It is not for us to create these healing substances. God did that already. It is for us to tune in with his wisdom and his will and to educate ourselves in how to restore our wellness and maintain our health by the use of his natural creations. Among these divine gifts are the oils of plants. God made them and gave us the intelligence to discover and learn how to use them.

This book is based on both scripture and science. It is a resource and a reference book wherein the ancient and Biblical arts of healing are related to the medical sciences of today. It is not the intent of this book to diagnose, prescribe, make medical claims, to practice medicine in any form, or to encourage anyone else to do so unless they are properly licensed to perform such functions. For these things you need to see a physician or other appropriate licensed health care professional.

Healing is a holistic spiritual term, not a medical one. The ancient priests and prophets, as well as some physicians of the *Bible*, anointed people with oil and prayed with them for their spiritual purification, moral repentance, and healing. So did Jesus. So did his disciples. And so did the Christians of the early church.

What Are Healing Oils?

The healing oils of the *Bible* are all essential or aromatic. These oils are the vital fluids of plants that are their life blood. They are called "essential" because they are necessary for the life of the plant and contain the "essence" of the plant. Essential oils contain life force, intelligence, and vibrational energy that imbues them with healing power that works for people.

Essential oils are composed of tiny molecules that can penetrate into every cell, administering healing therapy at the most fundamental levels of our bodies. They differ from the fatty oils we use for cooking. Fatty oils are composed of molecules much too large to penetrate to cellular levels. The familiar vegetable oils we use for foods have no therapeutic powers, at least not in the same ways as essential oils.

Essential oils were inhaled, applied to the body, and taken internally by the peoples of Biblical times. Their benefits extend to every aspect of our beings: physical, emotional, mental, and spiritual. The ancient people of the Holy Land seemed to understand this quite well. They used aromatic oils for every purpose from maintaining wellness, to physical healing, to enhancement of spiritual states in worship, to emotional cleansing, to purification from sin.

The medicines manufactured by man cannot compare with the healing capabilities of essential oils. Man-made pharmaceuticals lack the life force, the intelligence, and the vibrational energy found in healing oils. Synthetic prescriptions all have undesirable side effects even when taken according to a doctor's directions. Some side effects can be deadly. No drug is capable of true healing. Furthermore, when more than one drug is taken at once, they work in disharmony. Dangerous inter-reactions can occur. Tens of thousands of people die every year from prescription medicines, not because they overdosed or failed to follow directions, but because such drugs are inherently dangerous. That is why only licensed doctors are allowed to prescribe them. Meanwhile, people on drugs are not cured. Instead, they find themselves trapped in a life-long dependency on drug companies and the health care system.

Compare this with essential oils. They have no serious side effects—none that are deadly. They can and do effect true healings. When more than one is used at once, they work in harmony. Dangerous inter-reactions do not occur. No one has ever died from a properly applied essential oil. They are inherently safe. That is why anyone can use them without the supervision or prescription of a doctor. Meanwhile, people with chronic diseases are cured and no longer need oils or any other medicine. They become free and are no longer dependent on the medical system.

We shall discuss these points at greater depth later in this book. The point here is that essential oils are a gift from God to us, his children. They are special. They have been a gift too long ignored and misunderstood. The time has come to correct those misunderstandings and bring essential oils back into the uses for which God intended them.

What Makes Essential Oils Special?

"In the beginning was the Word, and the Word was with God, and the Word was God." Thus begins the Gospel of Saint John. The creation story of Genesis begins with the statement: "In the beginning God created the heaven and the earth." Following that we find God speaking his creation into existence by his very Word. "And God said, Let there be light . . .And God said, Let there be a firmament . . .And God said, Let the earth bring forth grass, the herb yielding seed, and the fruit tree yielding fruit after his kind, whose seed is in itself, upon the earth: and it was so." We find the phrase, "And God said . . ." nine times in the first chapter of Genesis.

Word is a vibration, a frequency, a consciousness, an expression of energy. When God created the plants by his speaking voice, he imbued them with his Word and his intelligence. This includes the oils of the plants which he intended, from their very creation, to become our medicines when we need healing.

That is what is so special about essential oils. They contain power from God's Word. Artificial medicines, made by humans, contain no such power. That's why they cannot heal and never will. But, again, we shall discuss this in more detail in another chapter.

The point here is that essential oils are divinely ordained as medicines for God's children and are meant to be used with God's guidance, accompanied with prayer.

Essential Oils Held in High Esteem

In Philippians 4:18, St. Paul refers to "a fragrant offering" as an acceptable gift "and pleasing to God," which is a reference to the aromas of the essential oils used in the incenses, anointing oils, and sacrifices of worship among Jews and early Christians. For thousands of years, from the ancient Egyptians to the Israelites to the early Christians, frankincense has been widely used in worship, as well as a cure-all for disease. The odor of frankincense is spiritually uplifting, invoking a calm, prayerful, meditative state of mind. Frankincense was used daily in the synagogues and places of early Christian worship and is still burned or diffused in Catholic churches today.

In II Corinthians 2:15-16, St. Paul describes devout Christians as "sweet savors," "fragrances," or "aromas" spreading the Gospel "among the perishing," while, in Ephesians 5:2, he admonishes his fellow Christians to be imitators of Christ "who gave himself up for us, a fragrant offering and sacrifice to God."

The odors of aromatic oils must have been held in very great esteem by early Christians. Why else would St. Paul choose to compare them, not only as a metaphor for the qualities of a good Christian, but to the essence of Christ, himself?

Daily applications of essential oils in Biblical times were extensive, indeed. Seventy percent of the books of the *Bible* mention essential oils, their uses, and/or the plants from which they are derived. Chapter Five of this book tabulates 1,035 such references involving 33 species of aromatic herbs and trees.

The Holy Land: Crossroads of the World

It is not surprising that fragrant oils were a treasured and daily part of the lives of those who lived in the Holy Land during Biblical times. The strip of territory between the Mediterranean Sea and the Jordan River was the crossroads of trade for spices, oils, and aromatic herbs from throughout the known world of that day. While the region of Palestine is especially blessed with many indigenous plants that produce healing oils, it was also the junction of the major highways of traffic from north, south, east, and west. Appropriately, the very first reference to healing oils in the *Bible* is in Genesis 37:25 where a caravan of camels came by Jacob's flocks on its way from Gilead "bearing spicery and balm and myrrh, going to carry it down to Egypt."

Because of its strategic location for the international commerce of its day, the peoples of the *Bible* had access to a greater variety of essential oils, medicinal herbs, perfumes, and ointments than, perhaps, any of the other nations of that time. The *Bible* mentions oils and fragrances used by the Israelites and early Christians that came, not only from neighboring regions such as Arabia, Lebanon, Persia, Babylon, Southeastern Europe, Egypt, Libya, and other parts of Africa, but from as far as India, the Himalayas, Indonesia, and, perhaps, even China. The books by Anderson, Tisserand, and Watt, listed in the bibliography, are good sources for such information.

Oil in the House of the Wise

In Genesis 1:29-30, God gives to mankind every plant and tree for "food" (or "meat"). The actual Hebrew word translated as food (or meat) is "oklah," which literally means, "that which is eaten," which can include not only that which is consumed for caloric needs and daily nourishment, but also for medicines.

In Ezekiel 47:12 we read, "On the banks, on both sides of the river, there will grow all kinds of trees for food. Their leaves will not wither nor their fruit fail, but they will bear fresh fruit every month, because the water for them flows from the sanctuary. Their fruit will be for food and their leaves for healing." (NRSV) or "...Their fruit shall be for meat and their leaf thereof for medicine." (KJV) Similarly, we read in Revelation 22:2, "The leaves of the tree are for the healing of the nations."

In Proverbs 21:20 it states that "Precious treasure and oil remain in the house of the wise." (NRSV) or "There is treasure to be desired and oil in the dwelling of the wise." (KJV) Oils, of course, are extracts of the essential lipid-soluble fluids of plants which have both nutritional and healing properties as well as other uses. As you will discover through this book, keeping a supply of oils in your house is a wise thing to do, indeed.

It is clear from the *Bible* that God intended that the oils of plants be used for many purposes. The fatty oils, such as olive, almond, and flaxseed, served as food and fuel for light for the peoples of Biblical times. The aromatic or essential oils served for flavorings, perfumes, incense, anointing, burial, and embalming. Essential oils were also applied for emotional release, mental clearing, spiritual upliftment, physical healing, and prevention of disease. (The differences between essential and fatty oils are discussed in Chapter 2.)

A Bible Oils Program You Can Do

You can read this book through from front to back, but it is not necessarily designed to be read that way. This book is the outgrowth of a program on the "Healing Oils of the Bible" where we discuss some of the oils mentioned in scripture and pass them around the room as we speak. Chapter Fourteen (the last chapter) gives instructions for doing this program, while Appendices E and F provide pages you have permission to photocopy for handouts. (See p. 276)

This book is a resource for doing that program. It contains all the back-up research and background information you would ever need (and much more) to successfully do this program. One way to read this book is to go to Chapter Fourteen and read how to do the program, turning back to the appropriate resources as directed.

Another way to read this book is go to the table of contents and choose the titles that interest you most and read them first in any order you choose. Each individual chapter can stand alone as a complete writing by itself.

Another rewarding way to read this book is to gather the oils mentioned in Appendix E and sniff or anoint yourself with the oils as you encounter them in the text. When we mention galbanum, for example, you may want to open a bottle and smell the oil, noticing its fresh grassy fragrance. Then you may want to put a little on your forehead or your shoulders and see how it makes you feel grounded and close to mother earth. When you read the chapter on "Oils of Joy," you may want to apply some oil of Joy™.

Chapter Fourteen will teach you how to do the *Bible* Oils Program for groups in your community or, perhaps, for a friend or two around the kitchen table. We also advise you in that chapter how to approach pastors and churches to do the program in a sacred setting. Some tips on publicity are provided if you want to do a Bible Oils Program open to the public. A list of the oils and supplies needed for the program is given in the instructions, a list you may wish to consult now before reading further, in case you want to have the right oils handy as you read this book.

Which Version of the Bible to Use?

The primary and ultimate source of information for this book is the *Bible*, both *Old* and *New Testaments*. While we consulted several versions, the two most often quoted and used are the *Authorized King James Version* (KJV) first published in 1881 and the *New Revised Standard Version* (NRSV) published in 1989 by the National Council of the Churches of Christ. We also relied heavily on *Young's Analytical Concordance of the Bible* and *Strong's Exhaustive Concordance of the Bible*, which give the Hebrew and the Greek, with commentary, from which the English has been derived. Analysis of the languages in which the *Bible* was originally written led to many insights into the uses of essential oils in Biblical times not apparent from reading only the English translations.

We also relied heavily on *Harper's Bible Dictionary* and the excellent four-volume set, *The Interpreters Dictionary of the Bible*.

The *Authorized King James Version of the Bible* is, perhaps, not as accurate from a scholarly point of view but is the *Bible* most familiar to most Christians. It has a poetic and devotional quality not matched in other translations. That is why the KJV was chosen as the principal reference, despite its shortcomings.

The *New Revised Standard Version of the Bible* was our second source, which helps to place the information in this book in an up-to-date form, compatible with the latest scholarly translations. A variety of other translations, which are listed in the bibliography, were also consulted.

Of course, the KJV, as we know it, isn't the same one produced by King James and his committee of theologians in 1611. It is a revised and edited version published 270

years later. The original *King James Version* of 1611 contained the *Deuterocanonical* or so called *Old Testament
Apocrypha,* while the *Authorized* version of 1881, commonly used today, does not.

The Catholic Church has always accepted the
Apocryphal books as canonical. They are routinely published in the various Roman Catholic versions of the *Bible.*
The Protestant *Revised Standard Versions* of today also
include these books in their translations. However, the
usual copies of the RSV and NRSV available in Christian
bookstores do not include them unless one specially orders
copies that do.

The Apocryphal Old Testament

The *Old Testament Apocrypha* consists of fifteen books
written between 300 B.C. and 100 A.D. and covers Jewish
history and prophecy between the last book of the traditional *Old Testament* (Malachi) and the coming of Christ.
Whether inspired by God (and thus legitimate scripture to
be included with the *Bible*) or not—these books do offer
valid insights into the life of the Jews during the centuries
immediately before Christianity. Thus, they offer additional documentation as to the use of essential oils by God's
chosen people. We do not count the *Apocrypha* as a canonical part of the *Bible* in this book, but we did search these
books for references to essential oils. The results are tabulated in Appendix B.

There is also a collection of writings called the *New
Testament Apocrypha.* But we did not consider them for
this work. None of them have been accepted as canonical
by any church or ecclesiastical authority.

We did, however, look into the *Pseudepigraphal* books
which were written between 200 B.C. and 600 A.D. These
works are attributed to *Old Testament* authors, such as
Adam and Eve, Ezekiel, Solomon, and Enoch, the eighth
descendant of Adam and the father of Methuselah. While
obviously not very helpful in gaining new information
about the ancient times to which they were attributed,

they are helpful in understanding the general philosophy and thinking of the Jews during the period when the books were written. For example, certain teachings that were supposed to be kept secret are discussed in the *Pseudepigrapha*. (St. Paul's comment on the "third heaven" in II Corinthians 12:2-4 was one of those teachings.) You can read more on this in Appendix E entitled "Seventh Heaven."

Why I Wrote This Book

In 1956 I suffered a back injury that caused me chronic and severe pain for the next 43 years. I have always believed that God was the only source of true healing and I had prayed for relief many times. But my back pain continued and gradually got worse.

During 1999 my wife, Lee, and I took up the study of essential oils because we had heard that they were effective with many conditions and diseases. We were also aware of the *Biblical* references in Mark and James where healings took place with prayer, laying on of hands, and anointment with oils. We attended various training seminars and read many books. We were also introduced to the many *Bible* references to healing oils such as aloes, cassia, cypress, galbanum, frankincense, cedarwood, spikenard, and myrrh. We learned that the *Biblical* meaning of the word "anoint" means "to massage or rub with oil" and that the oils used for anointing in Biblical times were either pure essential oils or fatty oils (such as almond or olive) that contained essential oils.

By that time my back problem had worsened to the point that I could not lift heavy loads. I could not even lean over a bathroom sink to brush my teeth without the possibility of triggering painful muscle seizures that would require a visit to a chiropractor for relief. I could not sleep more than three hours in a bed without waking in pain. I would get up, walk around, and then sit in a reclining chair to sleep a couple of hours, only to wake up again. For years my nights had been spent between a bed and a chair.

I had received numerous chiropractic adjustments during those 43 years and always got relief, but only temporary. The allopaths (MDs) could offer nothing but narcotics or surgery, which I refused. I lived daily with a nagging back ache that varied from bearable to unbearable, but never completely went away.

At a seminar in September of 1999 we learned a method of prayerfully anointing with oils on the back and feet that often produced dramatic results. The procedure takes about an hour and has been given the name "Raindrop Technique." When we got home from the training, Lee anointed me. That very night I went to sleep and didn't wake up the entire night for the first time in years. My back was pain free. I had been healed instantly, completely, and permanently. God's healing power, facilitated through my faith, my wife's healing touch, and the oils God had created, had corrected the errors in the cellular memory of my back muscles and spine that had caused them to spasm and stay in misalignment all of those years. Ever since then, I have been able to carry heavy loads, move pianos and refrigerators, and do what strong men are supposed to do with no strain and no pain. I have the back of a young man again.

That inspired me to study the scriptures in depth, as well as the biochemistry of the oils. I began doing public programs on the *Healing Oils of the Bible*, passing around the oils for people to anoint themselves as we read the *Bible* verses that mentioned them. I witnessed many miracles at these programs. It was in praying, preparing, and producing these programs that I came to realize that God and Christ were guiding me to write a book to help restore to the Christian church its proper place in the healing of the sick and infirmed. I spent two years gathering material specifically for this book and spent only six months in the actual writing, but it has taken all of my life to gather and assimilate what is contained here.

That is how and why I wrote this book. I have seen and experienced miraculous healings through God's grace and through the vehicle of the healing oils he lovingly created for our use. I want everyone to receive such miracles.

The Mission of This Book

With the birth and development of the scientific method that began some five or six hundred years ago, people began to look for answers to life's deepest questions outside of the church. Their faith, which had been in God and the scriptures, was gradually transferred to secular agents and agencies. People came to believe that most, if not all, of life's answers could be realized by secular science. The very word "secular" means "against or outside of God."

Such belief has created an unfortunate dichotomy that separates the church from its rightful mission to heal. The majority of people today believe that you go to church to worship, to be saved, to pray, take communion, to bring your soul closer to God, to seek the company of spiritual companions, to attend potluck suppers, to enjoy church socials, to study the *Bible*, and myriads of other things. But when most people are sick, they don't go to church to be anointed and healed, as Christians once did. They go to doctors or hospitals or purchase an over-the-counter medication. I ask you: Can a system that delivers services under the name of "health care" really deliver health when it fails to acknowledge the very source from which flows all of life and vitality?

The sun is the sole source of sunshine whether we believe in it or not. God is the sole source of healing whether we realize it or not. We hope this book will be a step in the direction of restoring to the church its proper place in the healing of the sick, a role that has, in modern times, been secularized and lost.

David Stewart, Ph.D., R.A.
Marble Hill, Missouri
March 7, 2004

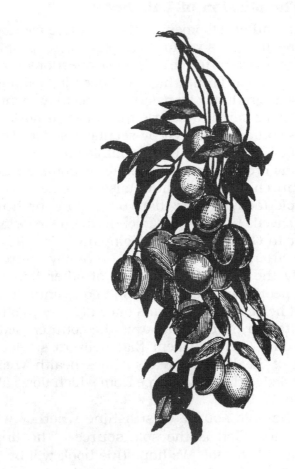

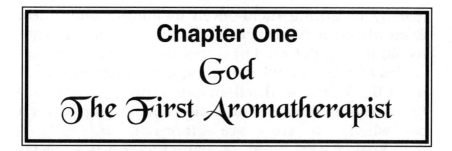

Chapter One
God
The First Aromatherapist

The story of oils in the *Bible* begins with Adam and Eve, when God placed them in a garden and not in a house. In Genesis, when God provided for all of their needs in that first paradise, there is no mention of a shelter of any kind. Instead, God placed them out-of-doors in a natural setting among the flowers, shrubs, grasses, and trees as their furniture and dwelling place. (Genesis 2:8)

Among the pleasant, rejuvenating things we like most about being close to nature are the smells of plants—the perfume of the honeysuckle, the smell of fresh grass, or the soothing fragrance that wafts from the needles and bark of cedar, juniper, spruce, and fir. All of these aromas come from essential oils, broadcast by plants as their means of communication between themselves, the animal kingdom, and people. Perhaps a lesson to be learned from the story of creation in Genesis is that God intended that we live in an environment permeated with the gentle scents of essential oils.

Scientifically, we now know that these natural aromas are more than just pleasant. They are emotionally, spiritually, mentally, and physically healing. God has imbued the aromatic molecules of plants, not only with the power to heal us when we are ill, but to nurture and preserve our health when we are well just by breathing them—even in minute quantities. Even when the fragrances of the flowers and trees are too faint to be detected by our sense of smell, the molecules of oils are still in the air, administering therapy to us. When we dwell among nature, we are continuously inhaling essential oils, twenty-four hours a day, whether we are aware of it or not.

In Ezekiel 47:12 and Revelation 22.2 it is suggested that God gave us the natural herbs, including their extracts, to be our medicines. Inasmuch as the science and art of aromatherapy is the inhalation, application, and ingestion of essential oils for healing and wellness, it appears that God was the first aromatherapist—long before the word or concept was articulated by humans.

Creating Your Own Eden

Now I am not suggesting that we all move out of our comfortable homes and sheltered workplaces and return to nature like Adam and Eve. Personally, I like living with heat in the winter, air conditioning in the summer, and shelter from the rain and wind. I don't think God has any problem with us living in the protected environments we have built for ourselves.

But there are some important implications in the *Bible* account of creation that place the first man and woman in a garden and not in a shelter that would have isolated them from nature and its aromatic atmosphere.

Fortunately, we don't have to give up our civilized ways to re-establish an aromatic environment in which to live and breathe. By using and diffusing pure essential oils in our homes and businesses, and as we travel, we can create an atmosphere permeated with the healing oils of Eden and enjoy the advantages of modern technology as well.

The First Mention of Oils in the Bible

The first time specific essential oils are mentioned in the *Bible* is in Genesis 37:25 in the story of Joseph. Joseph was the youngest son of Jacob and the favorite of his father. His older brothers became jealous to the point of hatred. They eventually plotted to kill him and tell their father that he had been attacked by wild animals. An opportunity to carry out their plot came when the brothers were miles away from their father's tent tending his flocks. Young Joseph had been sent by Jacob to check on his brothers and report back home. (Genesis 37:12-22)

When Joseph arrived at Dothan, where his brothers were, they seized him and threw him into a pit. As they were considering how they would carry out the murder and what story they should fabricate for their father, a caravan of Midianite traders, on their way to Egypt, chanced by, carrying "spicery, balm and myrrh." Seeing an opportunity for profit, while still accomplishing their intent to rid themselves of Joseph, they sold him to the Midianites for 20 pieces of silver. In Egypt he was sold to Potiphar, an officer of the Pharaoh. This incident took place around 1730 B.C. Joseph was a young teenage boy at the time.

To make a long story short, (Genesis 37–50), Joseph eventually found favor with the Pharaoh and was elevated from a slave to a ruler of all of Egypt— second only to the Pharaoh himself (Genesis 41:37-45). He was specifically given authority over the treasury and all of the stores of food and grain in the Kingdom. It was a powerful position, indeed. Joseph was thirty years old at the time.

Shortly after Joseph had been promoted to the throne of Egypt a famine struck the land, including the land of the Israelites. Jacob sent his sons to Egypt to buy grain for food. When they approached the Egyptian authorities for permission to purchase produce, it was Joseph with whom they had to deal. He recognized them as the brothers who had sold him into slavery many years before, but they did not recognize him. They could not see that beneath the power and splendor of the Pharaoh's grainhouse superintendent was their lost little brother.

It is a beautiful story of love, repentance, and forgiveness, which we won't retell here. You can read it in Genesis. The point we want to make is that the second time essential oils are mentioned in the *Bible* is where the sons of Jacob bring them to Egypt as gifts.

"And their father Israel (Jacob) said unto them, . . take of the best fruits of the land in your vessels, and carry down the man (Joseph) a present, a little balm, and a little honey, spices, and myrrh, nuts, and almonds." (Genesis 43:11)

Thus, "balm, spices, and myrrh," the aromatic oils and herbs carried by the Midianite traders (Genesis 37:25) when they took Joseph to Egypt as a prisoner and a slave are the very same ones sent to him many years later by his father and delivered by his brothers when he was a king. (Genesis 43:11)

True Extent of Oil Usage in Bible Times

There is more to the references to oils in the story of Joseph than meets the eye. These two verses imply that Jacob, his family, and the other peoples of his time obviously knew how to use essential oils and must have had a store of them, including many more varieties than just myrrh and balm. These two verses are but the tip of an iceberg of the considerable extent to which essential oils were actually used in those times and places. Appendix C contains a tabulation of oils of used in Biblical times but not mentioned in the *Bible*.

The fact is that dozens of essential oils and aromatic plants were used by the people of the Middle East in Biblical times. While many are mentioned in the *Bible*, many others were not. We know this from Roman, Greek, Egyptian, Arabic, Persian, Babylonian, Sumerian, and other sources. They were a daily part of the lives of the Israelites, yet the *Bible* is incomplete and vague about their usage.

Their Intent Was to Record God's Word

The lack of detail on the oils of the *Bible* is primarily because it was not the intent of *Bible* writers to discuss oils, but to present an account of the relationship of their people with God in a historical context. Hence, the majority of Biblical references to oils are related to worship (as in Exodus) and quasi-religious ceremonies such as the anointing of kings (as found in Samuel, Kings, and Chronicles) or such as burial and embalming (as found in Genesis and the Gospels). They are also mentioned as items of tithing in Matthew and Luke.

Only occasionally does the *Bible* digress into the secular use of oils as perfumes and odors (as in Esther and the Song of Solomon) or as agents of healing (as in Numbers, Leviticus, Isaiah, Mark, John, and James). The emotionally uplifting effects of inhaling the fragrances of oils are alluded to in Psalms, Proverbs, Isaiah, and Hebrews, but not discussed. The spiritual attributes of oils are suggested in many places in the *Bible* (as in Corinthians, Philippians, Ephesians, and Revelation) but are not explained.

Some Biblical mentions of essential oil-producing plants, such as the mustard seed of Matthew, Mark, and Luke, are almost accidental as parts of a parable to make a moral or spiritual point. Obviously, when Jesus told the story of the mustard seed, it had to be an item familiar to all of his listeners or he would not have chosen it to make his point. Yet mustard seed, which was a common source of medicinal oil as well as a flavoring for foods, is not mentioned anywhere else in the *Bible*, common as its usage was.

Why Explain the Obvious?

This leads to another point. The lack of detail in the use of essential oils in the *Bible* is not only because the authors were focused on other purposes, but also because oils, in the forms of incense, perfumes, spices, ointments, and medicines, were so much a part of the lives of everyone that no explanations were necessary. Why bother to explain something in print to people who already knew about common things such as oils and how to use them?

It would be like reading a book on the church leaders and religious beliefs of 20th century America and searching it for references to the medicines, deodorants, and perfumes used by modern Christians. Aspirin was probably the most popular analgesic of that time. Yet, would a theological history of the 1900s mention aspirin? And if it did, as incidental to making a religious point, would it bother to explain its indication or use? Why explain something that everyone already knows about? Hence, such topics would be omitted entirely in an ecclesiastical treatise or, at most, only casually mentioned without explanation or commentary.

Such is our situation with the Biblical record of essential oils and how they were employed. They were simply not a central part of the message intended by the *Bible* writers, even though mentioned. And just as modern readers would need no explanation for aspirin, the readers of the scriptures, at the time they were published, would need no explanation of oils. Hence, we find ourselves trying to glean botanical-medical information from a theological-canonical text.

Nevertheless, the *Bible* contains 33 species and more than 500 references to essential oils and the aromatic plants from which they came. (See Appendix A and Chapter Five on "How Many Oils in the *Bible*?")

A Little Balm, Spices and Myrrh

The *King James Version* of Genesis mentions "balm, spices, and myrrh" in two places. The Balm of Gilead is discussed in detail in Chapter Seven.

As for spices, the Biblical term applies to oil, gums, and resins, as well as to whole dried spices, whose spicy essences were in the oils they contained. When the *Bible* refers to "spices" for burial, the term refers to oils, not the dried herbs we know as spices today. (I Chronicles 16:14; Mark 16:1; Luke 23:56; 24:1; and John 19:40) The "spices" of the *Bible* would rarely resemble the crushed, ground, and powdered versions we purchase in grocery stores today. In any case, it is the oil content of a spice that supplies its flavor and aroma.

As for the myrrh in these passages of Genesis, it was probably not true myrrh (*Commiphora myrrha*), inasmuch as that tree grows in southern Arabia and Africa and not in Gilead nor in the land of Jacob. Hence, it would not be likely that traders from the north would be bringing myrrh to a country like Egypt who was geographically south and next door to the source.

The term "myrrh" (or "mor" in Hebrew) was applied

by the people of Biblical times to a number of resin-producing desert trees and shrubs, which makes identification of Biblical plants difficult and sometimes impossible. Sometimes even balm was confused with myrrh, since both could be referred to simply as "resin" or "aromatic gum" as was also frankincense, galbanum, onycha, cistus, and shittim (also known as gum arabic). The *New Revised Standard Version* (NRSV) doesn't use the word myrrh in Genesis. It uses the words "gum" and "resin."

The *Bible* word from which the *King James Version* translated the word "myrrh, was not the Hebrew "mor." King James relied heavily on the fourth century Latin translation of the *Bible* by St. Jerome (The *Vulgate*) and not the more ancient texts in Hebrew. In the *Vulgate*, the word in Latin was "labdanum" which can mean "myrrh." But in the original Hebrew the word was "lot" which is the resinous Rose of Sharon (*Cistus ladanifer*), also called "rock rose" or "cistus." Rock rose produces a medicinal resin and oil with some of the same properties as true myrrh.

It should be pointed out that throughout history oil of myrrh has been often mixed with other oils because of its unique ability to preserve fragrances and potency and make them last longer. Therefore, it is possible that the oil carried by the Midianites, though most likely the oil of the Rose of Sharon, also contained myrrh as a fixative. So King James' reference to myrrh would not necessarily be incorrect. What the Midianites carried may well have been a mixture of cistus and myrrh.

These points illustrate the difficulty in identifying oils and their species throughout the *Bible*. We shall discuss myrrh at greater length in the chapter entitled "Myrrh: The Most Popular Oil of the *Bible*." The Rose of Sharon is discussed in the chapter entitled "Roses of the Holy Land."

Essential Oils from Birth to Death

The beginning of Genesis tells the story of creation and how God placed the first man and woman in a garden where they would live and breathe the oils of plants gently floating in the atmosphere continuously night and day. This suggests that God's original plan was that his children be in contact with essential oils—living and breathing in their presence throughout life.

The end of Genesis refers to essential oils in yet a different context—their use in death. When Joseph was reunited with his family he gave them a place to live in Egypt in the Land of Goshen. When his father, Jacob (or Israel) died, Joseph had him treated like royalty and embalmed. (Genesis 50:2) The Egyptian embalming process for important persons, such as the father of a ruler like Joseph, was to employ a variety of essential oils. These would always include cedarwood, frankincense, and myrrh. Other oils known to have been used for embalming by the Egyptians included rosemary, juniper and cinnamon, but it seems that cedarwood, frankincense, and myrrh were always used at the time of Jacob and Joseph. In *New Testament* times, sandalwood (aloes) was another burial oil in common usage. (John 19:39) Basil was another burial oil in Jesus' day, but not in Jacob's time. The embalming process, carried out on Jacob's body by Egyptian physicians, took forty days.

While the first verses of Genesis concern a perfect garden for Adam and Eve to dwell among the fragrances of nature, the very last verse of Genesis

(Genesis 50:26) involves the fragrances of natural oils following the death of Joseph the Egyptian ruler as they prepared his body for burial.

> "And Joseph died, being 110 years old. He was embalmed and placed in a coffin in Egypt."

Even the coffin was an application of natural fragrances, being, no doubt, fashioned from the aromatic wood of the Cedars of Lebanon as was the custom for Egyptian notables in that day. In addition to oils of frankincense, myrrh, and cedarwood applied directly to the body of Joseph—his very coffin was a diffuser of the oily vapors of cedarwood.

Chapter Two
How and Why Oils Can Heal

In addition to the essential oils of balm, spices, and myrrh, Jacob also sent the Egyptian Emperor some "nuts and almonds." (Genesis 43:11) The nuts would have included walnuts and pistachios, which, along with the almonds, were all sources of food oils for the Israelites.

Oils pressed from nuts or seeds, however, are not particularly aromatic. While healthful as foods and useful as bases for perfumed massage oils or oils for anointing, they do not have the healing properties as do the oils of spices and other fragrant plants. Thus we see that plants produce two kinds of oil: non-aromatic fatty oils and fragrant essential ones. All healing oils are aromatic. Here is why.

Oleo-Gum-Resins

Essential oils are found in the circulating juices of plants, which are technically called "oleo-gum-resins." Following strict scientific definitions for the term, the "resin" part of the fluid is alcohol soluble, from which medicinal tinctures can be obtained. Tincture of benzoin is one of these, derived from the oleo-gum-resin of onycha. (Exodus 30:34) In Biblical times the gum was sometimes extracted by the alcohol in wine. The Romans often added the oleo-gum-resin of myrrh to wine, which helped prevent it from vinegarizing (turning sour) and which also provided a narcotic to deaden pain. Wine laced with myrrh helped Roman soldiers endure the discomforts of military life such as cold damp nights on the ground. Such wine was also drunk by shepherds sleeping in the fields and was offered to Christ just before he was nailed to the cross. (Mark 15:23)

The "gum" part of the plant fluid is water soluble and was, in fact, extracted by soaking or boiling leaves, dried herbs, or flowers in water creating aqueous solutions such as rose water. Gums also contain the sugar, carbohydrate, amino acid, and protein portions of the plant fluid.

"Oleo" is the oil, or lipid-soluble, water-immiscible portion, of the plant fluid. In Biblical times the oleo was extracted in a variety of ways. (See Chapter Twelve on "Extracting Essences in Biblical Times.") When oils are extracted by steam distillation, the condensed vapors separate into oil and water. The watery portion of the distillate contains the water soluble ingredients of the plant fluid, as well as traces of emulsified oil. The resulting liquid also has healing and health benefits. These by-products of distillation are called floral waters, essential waters, or hydrosols, and were also available in Biblical times.

Crude Resins of Frankincense and Myrrh

For example, oils of frankincense and myrrh are extracted from their oleo-gum-resins, which are crude exudates from the bark of the tree. The oils of frankincense and myrrh are also present throughout their leaves, flowers, and branches, but these are not usually used as a source for the oil. The nomadic tribesmen of southern Arabia and northern Africa have historically burned frankincense and myrrh wood for cooking fires and warmth, thus receiving the beneficial vapors of these oils through the smoke. The composition of the oleo-gum-resins of these trees is approximately as follows: 60% gum, 35% resin, and 5% oil. Thus you can see that the extracted oil, in this case, would be 20 times more concentrated than the natural oleo-gum-resin. Both the distilled oil concentrates and the natural bark exudates have healing powers. Both were used in Biblical times.

As for proper use of the technical terms "oleo," "gum," and "resin," we shall not conform to their strict scientific definitions in this book. The botanists, historians, Biblical scholars, and encyclopedia writers whom we used as our sources of information on the plants of the Holy Land used the terms "resin" and "gum" as synonyms, representative of the whole crude exudate. They never used the term "oleo." We shall do the same.

Tap Into the Full Potential of Plants

It is important to mention here that alcohol tinctures and aqueous solutions from medicinal herbs also have God-given healing powers, but they are different than those of essential oil distillates. While the oil might be effective for one condition, the tinctures and solutions may be effective for others and may not be effective for the same conditions as the oil.

Dried herbs are concentrates of the non-volatile portions of plant fluids which become available for healing by applying them as poultices and by brewing them as various teas. The consumption of living herbs, fresh greens, and vegetables is yet another avenue of tapping into the healing capabilities of plants.

God's intent for us to use plants for our medicines (Ezekiel 47:12; Revelation 22:2) is more than just their oil. God's intent is for us to take responsibility for our own health care and use the intelligence he gave us, guided by Him through prayer. This is the way we can personally discover the medicines he created for us and how to use them. This is how we can alter our lifestyles to live free of disease—which is God's desire for us.

When we surrender our health care decisions entirely to professionals, whose training is in commercial medicines devised for profit and the maintenance of a secular system, we are not taking responsibility for our own health care. We are not following God's divine directions. By such surrender to secular medicine, we are abdicating our birth right to health and longevity.

If you misplace your reading glasses in the kitchen, it won't help to look for them in the living room. Scientific medicine does not have all the answers. In fact, if you truly want to be healed, well, and whole, they hardly have any of the answers—especially when it comes to chronic diseases. Looking for solutions to most disease conditions within the medical practices of today is like looking for something that isn't there. It's the wrong place. (Mark 5:25-26; Luke 8:43) If we restrict ourselves to what the medical community has to offer, most of the time we will have cut ourselves off from any hope of real healing. The cures for most illnesses don't exist within that system. But they do exist.

Pray and See Where God Leads

If one prays with an open mind, free of the influence of modern medical propaganda and pharmaceutical advertising, one will be led by God to consider "alternative medicine." You would be guided to step outside of today's medical conventions. Much of what is called "alternative medicine" in today's terminology is actually "original medicine"—that which was effective thousands of years ago but which has been forgotten (suppressed) and supplanted by the chemical/medical industry of modern times.

If you can clear yourself of the prejudices that modern health education may have planted in your mind by corporate medicine, and if you can pray and sincerely surrender to God, you will be guided to consider the entire spectrum of medicinal plant possibilities—fresh leaves, dried herbs, waters, tinctures, and oils. This book, however, is focused on the oils.

How and Why Essential Oils Heal

Essential oils (the oleo portion of the plant fluid) are chemically very special in the universe of God's natural substances. Whether used in a pure concentrated state, in the natural whole juice, in the fresh plant, dissolved in a fat, or as aromatic vapors inhaled in the air, their healing power has been known and used since the most ancient of times. This is testified in Egyptian hieroglyphics dating more than 5,000 years ago. They are considered to be the first medicines of mankind and were an important part of the prescriptions of Hippocrates, the famous Greek physician whose works were published around 400 B.C.

Essential oils are composed of tiny molecules, all less than 500 atomic mass units (amu) in molecular weight. By contrast, fatty oils are composed of much larger molecules, many weighing 1000 amu and more. This difference is crucial to understanding why essential oils heal and fatty oils do not, at least not in the same ways.

Because of their infinitesimal sizes, essential oil molecules can easily pass through all of the tissues of the plant and into their very cells, passing right through cell walls. Thus they bring nutrition and information into the cell and carry waste products out. The fact that they are oils (mixtures of lipid compounds) enhances this penetrating power enabling them to administer to the plant's needs from gross circulation to the internal workings of a cell.

Any essential oil placed anywhere on the body is transdermal and can reach every part of your body within minutes. Some people can put an oil, such as cinnamon, cassia, or peppermint, on the soles of their feet and taste it on their tongue in less than a minute. (CAUTION: Please don't put oils neat on sensitive areas of the skin. The bottoms of the feet are okay.)

Oils as Universal Medicines

In serving plant functions, essential oils perform many duties. They regulate plant growth, like hormones. They help in plant metabolism, like enzymes. They also provide the basis for the plant's immune system warding off undesirable viruses, bacteria, microbes, fungi, parasites, and insects. When a plant is cut, it bleeds the oleo-gum-resin into the wound which initiates healing.

Because God created the plants for us (Genesis 1:11-12, 28), their oils can serve many of the same purposes for us as they do in plants. Thus, they can support and balance our endocrine, circulatory, digestive, nervous, and reproductive systems. They can clear our sinuses and lungs to help us breathe better. They can help us metabolize our nutrients, minerals, and vitamins. They can also boost the natural defenses of our immune systems so we can fight off disease by our own abilities. And while they are friendly to us, they can be hostile to bacteria, viruses, parasites, and fungi. In this way they can attack invading offenders directly.

Many oils, applied to the skin, are also effective insect repellents. Cedarwood and myrrh are excellent in this regard, a fact that has been known and applied since ancient times. Citronella was also used as an insect repellent in Biblical times, but is not mentioned in the *Bible*. A few drops of mint, a Biblical oil, can be mixed with water and sprayed on rose bushes to control aphids.

And just as the bleeding resins of plants fill the wound and initiate the healing process for the plant, pouring of essential oils into cuts and wounds can accelerate healing and protect from infection because of their antiseptic capabilities. Most essential oils are microbicides to some extent. The most gentle Biblical oils are aloes (sandalwood), balm, bay, bdellium, coriander, cumin, frankincense, galbanum, henna, juniper, myrrh, onycha, rue, shittim (acacia), and spikenard. The stronger antiseptic Biblical oils include anise, calamus, cassia, cedarwood, cinnamon, cypress, dill, fir, hyssop, mint, mustard seed, pine, terebinth and wormwood.

Still More Healing Properties of Oils

As if the foregoing were not enough to demonstrate the amazing abundance of healing properties of essential oils, they are also the world's most powerful antioxidants that can gobble up free radicals in our bodies. Scientists at Tufts University have developed a scale for the U.S. Department of Agriculture called the ORAC test (ORAC = Oxygen Radical Absorption Capacity). The higher the ORAC score, the more capable that particular food or oil is of destroying free radicals, thus retarding the aging process and preventing cancers and other diseases. The lists on the next page give some examples of ORAC scores:

Antioxidant (ORAC) Scores
For Selected Fruits and Vegetables

Carrots	210
Oranges	750
Beets	840
Raspberries	1,220
Strawberries	1,540
Blueberries	2,400
Wolfberries	25,300

Antioxidant (ORAC) Scores
For Selected Essential Oils

Sandalwood (Aloes)	1,655
Juniper	2,517
Rosemary	3,309
Rose of Sharon (Cistus)	38,624
Cinnamon Bark	103,448
Thyme	159,590
Clove	10,786,875

All of the oils listed above were in use during Biblical times and all but Rosemary, Thyme, and Clove are mentioned in the *Bible* by name. The contrast in the two sets of figures is striking. Chinese wolfberries are the highest scoring food in the world while Clove is the highest scoring essential oil and is 400 times more potent as an antioxidant than wolfberries. Most essential oils score higher than most fruits and vegetables, as the two tables above suggest.

In fact, essential oils have the highest ORAC scores of all the substances in the world. An ounce of Clove Oil has the antioxidant capacity of 450 lbs of carrots, 120 quarts of blueberries or 48 gallons of beet juice.

While eating foods high in antioxidants is a desirable and very healthy thing to do, learning to use essential oils in your daily life can potentially be even more desirable and health producing. The exceptionally high ORAC scores of essential oils partially explains why living with them in your daily environment—to breathe, eat, and apply to your body—can support all of your systems and contribute effectively towards long healthful living, even when used in very small quantities, and even when only inhaling them.

Longevity was common in early *Old Testament* times. In the fifth chapter of Genesis we read about Adam who lived 930 years and Methuselah who lived to 969. Both were healthy throughout their long lives. Both begat many sons and daughters throughout the many centuries of their lifetimes. Perhaps essential oils played a role in their virile and vigorously long lives.

God's Intelligence in Oils

The beauty of oils as medicines is that they don't have negative side effects like the synthetic drugs and chemicals of modern pharmacology. For example, the tinctures of iodine, merthiolate, mercurochrome, and other antiseptics may be effective in killing organisms that could invade an open lesion, but they are toxic, destructive to human tissue, and retard healing.

Oils are not only just as effective in their antiseptic powers, they are non-toxic, harmless to human tissue, and promote healing. Because they are direct creations of God's word (Genesis 1:11-12), when properly applied in a prayerful way they possess the divine intelligence to know how to do what is beneficial and to avoid doing that which may bring harm.

The Truth About Antibiotics

When it comes to dealing with an illness of bacterial or viral origin, the antibiotics of doctors are totally ineffective against viruses (which are the causes of flus and the common cold). When they do what they are designed to do, that is, destroy pathogenic bacteria in our bodies, they also destroy the friendly bacteria that our bodies need to support metabolism and the immune functions of the body.

When we have recovered from an illness with the help of antibiotics, the invading organisms may have been destroyed, but our immune systems have also been depressed. This makes us more susceptible to the next invasion of a bacteria, fungus, or virus. Hence, when children start receiving antibiotics for ear infections and other ailments of childhood, they get caught in a descending spiral of ever-recurring sickness. Once they get over one illness, they are ripe for the next. When they are sick again their systems require stronger and stronger antibiotics until they eventually end up with some sort of chronic (and possibly serious) disease later in life. This is because prescription drugs, as flawed fabrications of man, are spiritually dead and devoid of divine intelligence to know how to do only the right thing, and not the wrong.

Smart Medicine

By contrast, when essential oils are used to attack a bacteria which has invaded our bodies, they are selective because they are imbued with God's intelligence. They know which are the bad guys and which are the good ones so that when they have killed off the bacteria causing the sickness, the good bacteria are still alive to serve us. Healing and dealing with bacterial illness with God's medicines leaves our immune systems stronger after the illness than before, thus working toward the prevention of future disease. This is quite unlike antibiotics that weaken us and encourage the contraction of future diseases.

We are not saying that antibiotics have no place in the healing arts. They do, but they should be used sparingly and with caution. Their side effects must be taken into account. Their long-term negative consequences may, in most cases, well outweigh any immediate temporary benefit. God created our bodies to fight off most infections. That's why he gave us immune systems. It is important not to take medicine (or any substance) that compromises the innate healing abilities God has given to us. God's medicines support our innate healing abilities. Seek the opinions of competent healing professionals who understand and accept God's role in healing in matters such as these.

Why Healing Oils are Fragrant

If you can't smell an oil at a distance, it probably isn't essential. Exceptions to this include some natural, volatile oils that have only faint fragrances not always perceptible to people. The healing oils of the *Bible* are all aromatic even when their aromas are not strong. That is to say, they are volatile and can be inhaled. We can't smell liquids or solids, only gases. Only molecules that can vaporize and leap into the atmosphere can enter the nose and be smelled.

Most essential oils are noticeably fragrant—some strongly so, some pleasant, and some not so pleasant. Some are only weakly detectable to the nose. In all cases, the oils do easily evaporate, which is because their molecules are small and energetic. Hence, the molecular property (small size) that enables them to penetrate human tissue and pass through cell membranes is also the property that makes it possible to smell them and take them into our bodies through the olfactory system. In so doing, the molecules not only reach all parts of the body via the blood stream accessed through our lungs, they also go directly to the brain, crossing the blood-brain barrier. Thus originates the term "aromatherapy" where essential oils can be applied for therapeutic purposes merely by inhaling or breathing in their aromas.

Two Kinds of Oils in Plants

Vegetable oils cannot enter the blood stream nor cross the blood-brain barrier. Their uses in aromatherapy are restricted to providing a neutral lipid base in which essential oils can be blended for massage or diluted when application of the pure concentrated oil may be too strong. The molecules of fatty oils are too large to evaporate and too large to penetrate cellular dimensions and circulate through the tissues of the body. While essential oils were created to circulate within a plant to carry out its functions as a living creation, fatty oils are manufactured in the seed where they remain uncirculated through the life of the plant.

This is as God intended. The heavy seed oils of a plant are for the future preservation of the species, not for the current life of the plant that produces them. To manufacture the sugars and starches that serve as food to the plant, it takes sunlight beaming on green stems and leaves containing chlorophyll, along with a root system to draw minerals and moisture from the earth. When a seed first germinates in the ground, it has no stem, leaves, or roots. So how is the budding new plant supposed to live until its food factory is ready for production?

The answer is in the fatty oil where just enough food has been provided to the new plant to live until it can make its own food. That is why God put the oil there and why it does not circulate. The fatty oil is an advance payment to the young plant until it can produce on its own—at which time the debt is paid back to God as a contribution to the next generation.

Most seeds also contain both fatty and essential oils. Biblical examples include anise, coriander, cumin, dill, and mustard. When the seeds are pressed to squeeze out their vegetable oils, the volatile essential oils usually evaporate, leaving the fatty oils behind. When seeds are steam distilled, only the lighter essential oils pass through the evaporation/condensation process leaving the fatty oils back in the plant mass in the cooker. In some cases, the leaves and stalks of a plant (such as dill) produce a different essential oil than the seeds. Hence, from the same plant source, both fatty and aromatic oils can be obtained, as well as more than one variety of the aromatic kind.

Some fatty oils, such as olive, contain aromatic molecules as well. The "beaten" oil of Biblical times was a blend of both types of oil. See Chapter Eleven entitled "Olive: The Other Healing Oil of the *Bible*."

The Sex Life of Plants

While fatty oils are placed in the plant to play a role in reproduction, essential oils also play a role in that regard as well. Plants use their odors to attract animals and insects by which they pollinate, an essential step in growing fertile seed for the continuation of the species. It is interesting to note that the strong attracting fragrances of some flowers disappear (sometimes within thirty minutes) once they have been pollinated. Hence, when extracting oils from flowers it is crucial to do so at the right time before the desired aromatic essential oil has been chemically altered and removed by the plant.

Of course, from time immemorial women have worn perfumes fashioned from the scents of leaves, roots, and flowers to attract men and make themselves appealing to the opposite sex. For example, Esther (2:12) applied oils of myrrh and other perfumes to her body for a whole year in preparation for her marriage to King Ahasuerus. King Solomon in his Song 4:9–16 sings of how his bride has "ravished his heart," and extols the "fragrances of the oils" of his beloved mentioning by name the perfumed oils of nard, henna (camphire), saffron, calamus, cinnamon, frankincense, myrrh, and aloes (sandalwood). Thus, we find many parallels between the ways in which essential oils serve both plants and people.

Oils and Emotions

One of the most powerful healing aspects of essential oils is their ability to penetrate the so called "Blood-Brain Barrier." When you breathe oil molecules into the back passages of your nose, they go straight to the brain in a central part called the amygdala (or diencephalon). This is the central headquarters of the limbic system, which manages your storage and filing system for all your emotional experiences. That part of the brain does not understand words and cannot be communicated to with spoken or written language. It responds only to smell. Hence, essential oils provide a powerful means to contact that non-verbal portion of our brains that stores our feelings and emotions.

This is why when you smell apple pie, for example, you may find yourself back in your grandmother's kitchen as a little child. That is why the smell of frankincense brings a Catholic back to the sanctuary where they went to church and inhaled that fragrance so many Sundays.

Bigger than All the Computers of the World

You will be interested to know that whereas the center of the brain is the coordinator of emotional memories, the memories are not actually stored there. That part of the brain performs the functions of a librarian who catalogues all the emotional memory books and then assigns a location on the shelves of your bodily temple to hold that information for future reference. When we have an emotional experience, especially a traumatic or painful one, the amygdala assigns a part of your body to remember that experience until you are ready to deal with it.

The body is composed of some 100 trillion cells each with a strand of DNA capable of storing up to six gigabytes of memory that can replicate RNA memory strands without limit. The emotional brain can delegate any place in your body to store a feeling or an emotional memory. You will never run out of memory storage space. What you carry in your body is greater than the combined memories of all the computers in the world. You and every other human being has this amazing capability.

If you think that the human species is the result of billions of years of chance evolution from the accidental juxtaposition of the elements, understanding the beautifully structured memory storage and retrieval system we each possess is more than sufficient to disprove such notions. Only a kind and benevolent God could conceive and create such elegant and complex sophistication and keep it working with no conscious thought on our parts.

Which of you by taking thought can add one cubit to his stature?
Matthew 6:27

How Emotions Can Make us Sick

When an essential oil penetrates into the central brain, it makes it possible for us to access forgotten memories of emotions with which we need to deal. Stored emotions can make us sick. If they are stored in the stomach, you can have stomach ailments. If in the pancreas, you can have diabetes. If in the liver, you can have many problems. If in the thyroid or other endocrine glands, you will have hormonal problems. If in the joints, you can have arthritis.

Stored emotions can cause cancer, too, which is why women, whose breasts are their physical expression of love and nurturing, often have breast cancer. In such cases, some emotional trauma has been repressed and stored in cellular memory that blocks a woman's natural ability to let love flow towards others and/or towards themselves.

Hence, when essential oils trigger an emotionally upsetting memory, it gives us an opportunity to deal with that emotion and release it from our systems, thereby affecting a healing. Sometimes this healing is instantaneous with the release of the emotion and sometimes it takes longer. In either case, a healing results.

The Blood-Brain Barrier

It was thought for years that the interstitial tissues of the brain served as a barrier to keep damaging substances from reaching the neurons of the brain and the cerebrospinal fluid. Instead of a barrier, it would be more accurate to consider it as a sieve or filter through which only molecules of a certain size or smaller can pass.

Most of the molecules of the substances used in chemotherapy are too large to pass through the blood-brain filter, which is why doctors say that chemotherapy doesn't work on brain cancer. Some of the smaller molecules get through, but not the whole suite of drugs intended.

Doctors don't know for sure, but it seems that in order to cross the blood-brain barrier, only molecules less than 800-1000 atomic mass units (amu) in molecular weight can get through. Lipid solubility seems to be another factor which facilitates passing through the blood-brain barrier. Water soluble molecules don't usually penetrate into brain tissue, even when very small. The molecules of essential oils are all not only small, but lipid soluble as well.

In fact, when it comes to essential oils, small molecules (less than 500 amu) are what they are made of. That is why they are aromatic. The only way for something to be aromatic is for the molecules to be so small that they readily leap into the air so they can enter our noses and be detected as odor and smell.

That is why oils for cooking or massage, such as corn, peanut, sesame seed, safflower, walnut, almond, canola, olive and other oils pressed from seeds are not aromatic. Sure, they have a smell, but you can't smell them across the room in minutes as one can when you opens a bottle of peppermint, hyssop, or cinnamon oil.

Essential oils of every species cross the blood-brain barrier. This makes them uniquely able to address disease, not only from a physical level, but from a more basic and fundamental level—that of the emotions which are often the root cause of physical illness.

A Quick Course in Chemistry

Because of the tiny molecular structure of the components of an essential oil, they are extremely concentrated. One drop contains approximately 40 million-trillion molecules. Numerically that is a 4 with 19 zeros after it:

40,000,000,000,000,000,000,000. We have 100 trillion cells in our bodies, and that's a lot. But one drop of essential oil contains enough molecules to cover every cell in our bodies with 40,000 molecules. Considering that it only takes one molecule of the right kind to open a receptor site and communicate with the DNA to alter cellular function, you can see why even inhaling a small amount of oil vapor can have profound effects on the body, brain, and emotions. Sometimes too many oil molecules overload the receptor sites, and they freeze up without responding at all, when a smaller amount would have been just right. This is why we say that when using oils, "sometimes less is better." Sometimes more is better, too. Knowing the difference is the art of aromatherapy.

Essential oils are mixtures of dozens, even hundreds, of constituents, all of which are composed of carbon and hydrogen and sometimes oxygen. All essential oils are principally composed of a class of organic compounds built of "isoprene units." An isoprene unit is a set of five connected carbon atoms with eight hydrogens attached. Their molecular weight is only 68 amu, which is very small, indeed.

Molecules built of isoprene units are all classified as "terpenes." Terpenes are what make essential oils unique in the world of natural substances.

Phenols and Phenylpropanoids

Phenols and Phenylpropanoids are compounds of carbon-ring molecules incorporating one isoprene unit. They are sometimes called hemiterpenes. There are dozens of varieties of phenylpropanoids. They are found in Clove (90%), Cassia (80%), Basil (75%), Cinnamon (73%), Oregano (60%), Anise (50%), and Peppermint (25%).

While they can create conditions where unfriendly viruses and bacteria cannot live, the most important function performed by phenylpropanoids is that they clean the receptor sites on the cells. Without clean receptor sites, cells cannot communicate, and the body malfunctions, resulting in sickness.

Monoterpenes

Monoterpenes are compounds of two isoprene units, which is ten carbon atoms and sixteen hydrogen atoms per molecule—molecular weight 136 amu. There are an estimated 2,000 varieties of monoterpenes.

Monoterpenes are found in most essential oils: Galbanum (80%), Angelica (73%), Hyssop (70%), Rose of Sharon (54%), Peppermint (45%), Juniper (42%), Frankincense (40%), Spruce (38%), Pine (30%), Cypress (28%), and Myrtle (25%).

While offering a variety of healing properties, the most important ability of the monoterpenes is that they can reprogram miswritten information in the cellular memory (DNA) (restoring God's image, Genesis 1:26) . With improper coding in cellular memory, cells malfunction and diseases result, including lethal ones, such as cancer.

Sesquiterpenes

Sesquiterpenes are compounds of three isoprene units, which is fifteen carbons and twenty-four hydrogens per molecule—molecular weight 204 amu. There are more than 10,000 kinds of sesquiterpenes.

Sesquiterpenes are the principal constituents of Cedarwood (98%), Vetiver (97%), Spikenard (93%), Sandalwood (Aloes) 90%, Black Pepper (74%), Patchouli (71%), Myrrh (62%), and Ginger (59%). They are also found in Galbanum, Onycha, and Frankincense (8%).

Sesquiterpene molecules deliver oxygen molecules to cells, like hemoglobin does in the blood. Sesquiterpenes can also erase or deprogram miswritten codes in celluar memory. Sesquiterpenes are thought to be especially effective in fighting cancer. The root problem with a cancer cell is that it contains misinformation, and sesquiterpenes can delete that garbled information. At the same time the oxygen carried by sesquiterpene molecules creates an environment where cancer cells can't reproduce. Hence, sesquiterpenes deliver cancer cells a double punch—one that disables their coded misbehavior and a second that stops their growth.

The American Medical Association (AMA) has said that if they could find an agent that would pass the blood-brain barrier, they would be able to find cures for ailments such as Lou Gehrig's disease, multiple sclerosis, Alzheimer's disease, and Parkinson's disease. Such agents already exist and have been available since Biblical times. The agents, of course, are essential oils—particularly those containing the brain oxygenating molecules of sesquiterpenes.

The Triple Whammy

The big triple punch combination of "PMS" (Phenylpropanoids, Monoterpenes, and Sesquiterpenes) found in essential oils is probably one of the major aspects responsible for the therapeutic power familiar to essential oil users. Many oils containing PMS have been found to be useful in addressing many illnesses, injuries, and disease conditions. One hypothesis is that this combination offers the following actions:

First, Cleanse Receptor Sites: Phenols and phenylpropanoids can act to clean receptor sites on the surfaces of cells. This allows the proper transfer of hormones, peptides, neurotransmitters, steroids, and other intracellular messengers.

Second, Deprogram Bad Information: Sesquiterpenes seem to work at a subcellular level by affecting membrane fluidity and facilitating oxygen transfer. Sesquiterpenes may also affect transport of material inside the cell. This allows for access to DNA and RNA which may offer a scientific basis for "deprograming or erasing the incorrect information from cellular memory" often referred to in holistic healing circles.

Third, Reprogram Correct Information: Monoterpenes, working at both subcellular and intracellular levels, protect against free radical damage and work within cells to produce properly programed strands of RNA and DNA. This helps insure proper cell-to-cell communication and maintain healthy bodily functions. Many refer to this as "reprogramming the cells."

These three classes of chemical components may be why essential oils sometimes affect a healing that is nearly instant and also permanent. What they simply do is to restore the body back to its natural state of balance and health at the most basic and fundamental levels within the cells. The generational curses mentioned in the *Bible* (Exodus 20:5, 34:7; Numbers 14:18; Deuteronomy 5:9) that come to us through the genes or our parents are not immutable and incurable, as modern medical doctors believe. These inherited conditions can be reprogramed in the DNA by the actions of essential oils combined with laying on of hands and prayerful intent. The Biblical oils all contain some, if not all, of these constituents. This is one secret to their amazing healing abilities. Science will, in time, produce additional clarification of these processes, but this is our understanding at this time.

So there you have it in a nutshell: The way the blood-brain barrier works and the biochemistry of one of the ways essential oils can help achieve a healing. For more on PMS anointing, see *The Chemistry of Essential Oils Made Simple*, mentioned at the end of this book.

Electromagnetic Frequency

There is another dimension to the healing powers of essential oils. This has to do with their electrical properties. All essential oils carry electrical charges, usually electrons or negative ions, which are healing and healthful. They are also energetic, generating nanovolts of electricity (billionths of a volt) at megahertz frequencies (that's in the radio frequency range or millions of cycles per second.)

These frequencies are measurable with properly designed instrumentation. Bruce Tainio of Tainio Technology in Cheny, Washington, has developed sensitive frequency meters to measure such energies. In a series of experiments conducted by Tainio, reported in the *Reference Guide to Essential Oils* published by Abundant Health, the following was found.

The frequencies of essential oils are between 52-320 MHz—the highest of all known substances. The highest is Rose Oil at 320 MHz. Lower frequency oils resonate with the bodily systems that have those frequencies, such as the bones and joints, and, thus, administer healing vibrations to those systems. When several oils are blended together, a fundamental frequency will emerge that may be higher or lower than many of its components.

By comparison, fresh herbs measure 20-27 MHz, dry herbs 12-22 MHz, and fresh produce 5-10 MHz. Processed or canned food measured zero. In other words, there is no life or life force in canned or processed foods. They contain chemical nutrition, but not the vital, electronic nutrition of live fresh foods.

Measurements on the human body found that a healthy person has a frequency around 62-68 MHz. When a person's frequency dips to 58 MHz, cold symptoms can manifest. Flu symptoms start at 57 MHz, Candida at 55 Mhz, and Epstein Barr syndrome at 52 MHz. Cancer can begin when the body falls below 42 MHz. The process of dying begins at 25 MHz and goes to zero at death.

In other experiments by Tainio, he measured the effects of coffee, finding that even holding a cup of coffee lowers one's bodily frequency by 8 MHz and that taking a sip can lower one's frequency by 14 MHz. When essential oils are inhaled following the exposure to coffee, the bodily frequencies restore themselves in less than a minute, but if no oils are administered, it can take up to three days for the body to recover from even one drink of coffee.

Frequency data are not yet available on most oils. The table that follows gives a sample of electromagnetic frequencies for a few oils for which measurements have been made and published. (See *Reference Guide to Essential Oils* published by Abundant Health.)

Electromagnetic Frequencies
of Selected Oils

Rose (Rosa damascena)	320 MHz
Helichrysum (Helichrysum Italicum)	181 MHz
Ravensara (Ravensara aromatica)	134 MHz
Lavender (Lavendula angustifolia)	118 MHz
Blue Tansy (Tanacetum annum)	105 MHz.
German Chamomile (Matricaria recutita)	105 MHz
Melissa (Melissa officinalis)	102 MHz
Juniper (Juniperus osteosperma)	98 MHz
Angelica (Angelica archangelica)	85 MHz
Peppermint (Mentha piperita)	78 MHz
Galbanum (Ferula Gummosa)	56 MHz
Basil (Ocimum basilicum)	52 MHz

One of the most important healing modalities of the oils is their ability to lift our bodily frequencies to levels where disease cannot exist.

The Power of Prayer

Tainio also found that the frequencies of oils are also affected by thoughts. Negative thoughts lowered the frequencies of the oils by 12 MHz while positive thoughts raised them by 10 MHz. Prayer made an even greater difference, raising the frequency levels by 15 MHz.

This is important information. It has always been known that applying and receiving essential oils in an attitude of prayer greatly enhances their effectiveness. The above data offer a scientific explanation of why.

The point is that the Biblical application of essential oils was always with prayer. Sometimes prayer alone will work and sometimes oils alone will work, but the combination is very powerful, indeed. The intent and righteousness of the person applying the oil, as well as the faith of the receiver, has a great deal to do with the prognosis for success in healing. We must not only be intelligent and loving practitioners of aromatherapy, we must also live pure lives so that we may be clear channels for God's healing power. In Deuteronomy 7:13 Moses comments that God will bless the oil of a righteous person. Science has now found this to literally be true.

Six Ways that Essential Oils Support Us

(1) As fighters against unfriendly microbes.
(2) As balancers of bodily functions.
(3) As raisers of our bodily frequencies.
(4) As antioxidants that purify our systems.
(5) As clearers of negative emotional baggage.
(6) As uplifters of our spiritual awareness.

In these ways, the healing oils of the *Bible* accomplish their work by the innate therapeutic powers with which God has endowed them. But their greatest effectiveness is in combination with prayer, with which they were intended to be used.

Books on Healing with Oils

• For information on anointing with oils for healing combined with prayer, as well as a thorough discussion of the science and individual properties of essential oils, see *Healing Oils Healing Hands* by Linda L. Smith, RN, MS, CHTP.

• For detailed information on the use of oils for healing purposes, with applications to specific disease conditions, see the *Essential Oils Desk Reference*, edited by Brian Manwaring, *Essential Oils Integrative Medical Guide* by Dr. Gary Young (ND), or the *Reference Guide for Essential Oils* by Connie and Alan Higley.

• For information using oils for emotional releasing, see *Releasing Emotional Patterns with Essential Oils* by Dr. Carolyn Mein (DC).

• For information on the scriptural basis for healing to take place in a church setting, including anointment with oils, see *The Miracle of Healing in Your Church Today* by Rev. Jim Lynn. Care Publications also carries a two-hour video by Rev. Lynn of the same title.

• For a view of aromatherapy from a clinical perspective, see *Aromatherapy for Health Professionals* by Shirley and Len Price, *Natural Home Health Care Using Essential Oils* by Daniel (MD) and Rose-Marie Penoel or *Medical Aromatherapy* by Kurt Schnaubelt (PhD).

• For a medical doctor's viewpoint with a historical perspective, as expressed by one of the early pioneers, see *The Practice of Aromatherapy* by Jean Valnet, MD.

• For an easy-to-understand scientific explanation of how essential oils work, presented in a scriptural context, see *The Chemistry of Essential Oils Made Simple* by David Stewart. (see p. 324)

• All of these books are listed in the Bibliography. Most bookstores can order them for you. You may also contact the publisher of this book for information on how to obtain them. Several titles mentioned above are carried by Essential Science Publishing, Abundant Health, and others. Besides bookstores, many of these books are also obtainable from the website, www.RaindropTraining.com.

Chapter Three
Atheistic Medicine and The Priesthood of Healing

In ancient cultures the world over, the healers of a society were also the priests. With the advent of science a few centuries ago, men's faith in God began to be replaced by faith in science in the belief that the scientific method could provide answers to all of life's questions. With that came the development of secular or atheistic medicine, which is what professional health care has become today.

Now I am not saying that doctors and nurses are atheists. I am saying that the text books of medicine and nursing are devoid of acknowledgement of God as the ultimate and sole source of healing. Prayer and God communion are not required disciplines in medical or nursing schools anywhere.

The False God of Our Times

It is now apparent that the secularization of the healing arts has been a major error leading to countless deaths and the destruction of personal wellness. While science has served us well in improving our standards of living and bringing us many advances, people have grown to expect more from science than science can possibly deliver. It has become a false god, the idol of modern civilization. The scientific method cannot touch the most important aspects of our existence and will never have the answers for most of life's important questions.

The worship of science is particularly manifest with modern medicine in which people have come to place more faith than they have in God and Christ. This includes most church-going Christians. The book, *Confessions of a Medical Heretic*, by physician, Robert S. Mendelsohn, M.D., listed in the bibliography, describes how people have come to regard modern medicine with a faith traditionally reserved for religion. According to Mendelsohn, doctors are regarded as priests, and hospitals are regarded as temples where medical miracles take place in response to the dispensing of holy waters (drugs, serums, and antibiotics, etc.) and the performance of rituals and sacrifices (surgery and radiation). Furthermore, the public is coerced into "tithing" to the health care system through insurance and tax-supported medical programs, where the amount of the tithe is not a mere 10%—but 20% of one's income and more.

We read of the idols and false gods of the *Old Testament* and smile because we see them for what they are. We wonder how large numbers of intelligent people could have believed in inanimate objects as having life and divinity. We can't believe how *Old Testament* idol worshippers could have placed their faith and their very lives on such a transparently false basis. But idols and false gods are just as abundant today as they ever were and millions bet their lives on them. The principal idol most people worship today is allopathic medicine, which appears legitimate and real because it wears the mask of science.

Cures vs. Management

According to Dr. Mendelsohn, today's system of "health care" is really "sick care," health being outside the domain of medicine. "The best of medicine is emergency medicine," says Mendelsohn, "when there is a real crisis to deal with." As for chronic disease and the common flus and colds (which represent 95% of the conditions people suffer), modern medicine has no cures, only treatments that never end. The hidden objective of today's medical profession is to generate as much repeat business as possible. They don't aim to cure. Cured people don't come back, only the sick. A healthy population is bad business for the medical system.

I am sure that if they were aware of cures, most physicians would prescribe them. But for most conditions, they have no cures within the confines of their allopathic education. They have treatments, but not cures. Essential oils, which can lead to complete healing, are not within their paradigm.

In place of a cure, most doctors will just try to manage your sickness. If they follow the protocols and standards by which they are pledged to practice, they will eventually place you on a regimen of life-long dependency and turn you into a life-long source of income for themselves and the system they serve.

Doctors are also good at taking a simple issue and escalating it into an acute problem through their interventions. They can transform a simple condition into a life threatening crises. They may not be able to correct minor ailments, but serious problems they can handle. Such is their training.

When I was in medical school, an obstetrics professor once told a class of medical students, where I was present, that to him normal labor was boring, but doing cesarean surgery was exciting. "It makes your day," he commented. As a result of such teachings and attitudes, six out of seven cesareans today are unnecessary and do far more harm than good.

Doctors love to practice heroic medicine. Dr. Mendelsohn likens them to firemen fighting to rescue the perishing by putting out fires that they started. In the process, people die unnecessarily. Survivors rarely realize that the cause of their loved one's demise was the system from which they had sought help.

Hippocrates, the father of physicians, required an oath of his students that started, "*primum no nocere*," "First do no harm." That oath is not taken by physicians any more. It hasn't been a part of medicine for more than half a century. A God-based medical system would do no harm, but the pharmaceutically based system that has control over health care today does a great deal of harm. The numbers are staggering.

A Passenger Jet Crash Every Day

According to the U.S. Centers for Disease Control and Prevention (CDCP) over the past decade, more than two million people are admitted to hospital emergency rooms each year suffering from adverse drug reactions from prescriptions or over-the-counter medications. More than 100,000 people die every year in the United States from properly administered prescription drugs. At least another 100,000 die from improperly administered drugs and other medical mistakes. Deaths caused by physicians are called "iatrogenic." Deaths due to hospital-caused factors are called "nosocomial." The CDCP has a whole division for the tabulation and study of iatrogenic and nosocomial deaths and diseases.

The July, 2000, issue of the *Journal of the American Medical Association*, attributes 250,000 deaths a year to doctors and pharmaceuticals with prescription drugs as the third leading cause of death in the United States and iatrogenia (doctor mistakes) as the eighth.(See www.mercola.com).

250,000 iatrogenic fatalities per year is many times more than those who die from illegal drugs. Yet if a couple of dozen people die from street drugs in a month's time in a given area, that becomes national news. Yes, we have an illegal drug problem in America, but it pales when compared to the problem of legal medicine legally administered.

250,000 iatrogenic deaths a year comes down to 5,000 deaths a week. That is equivalent to a jumbo jet crashing every day killing all the passengers and crew. Even one such crash is cause for national mourning. Such tragedies spawn news stories for weeks to follow and prompt immediate and thorough investigations. But nothing is ever said in the news about an even worse tragedy happening every week, month after month, year after year, for decades. Even though the U.S. Centers for Disease Control routinely tabulate and publish the damaging data, there are no federal or congressional investigations that lead to an alleviation of the problem. This is what atheistic medicine does.

How Many People Die from Herbs and Oils?

Dr. Kurt Schnaubelt (Ph.D.) in his book, *Advanced Aromatherapy*, states that "the American Association of Poison Control Centers reported 809 fatal poisonings and 6,407 serious but non-fatal poisonings from conventional pharmaceuticals between 1988 and 1989, whereas "Plant-based preparations caused two fatalities and 53 serious poisonings in the same time period. The most dangerous plants were not medicinal. They were house plants and shrubs." In the same time frame, there were no serious or fatal poisonings from essential oils.

According to a 2002 article entitled "The Science of

Deceit" by Burton Goldberg found on the web page <www.alternative medicine.com>, "Mainstream media regularly reports on the 'dangers' of 'unproven' herbal remedies and supplements. But what is the reported number of people who have actually died from using herbs and supplements? According to the FDA, in the five year period between 1993 and 1998, federal, state, and local agencies reported only 184 such deaths—most of which were associated with weight loss formulas."

As for deaths by essential oils, the only recorded cases appear to be in England with only five or six instances in the last one-hundred years. A couple of these fatal incidents involved unsupervised young children who managed to swallow an ounce or two of essential oil all at once. Other cases involved women seeking to abort their babies by drinking large quantities of wormwood or other strong essential oils, causing their own death as well as that of the fetus.

There has never been a case recorded anywhere of anyone dying from an essential oil administered by a qualified aromatherapist or taken according to common sense precautions.

Compare this with the 200,000 thousand plus people who die in America every year from physician administered drugs and procedures. During the same period of time (1993-98) when fewer than 200 deaths occurred from herbs and supplements, almost a million people died from FDA-approved, properly prescribed, medically administered pharmaceuticals and medical procedures. Iatrogenia has become a leading cause of death in the United States, only slightly behind cancer and cardiovascular disease.

Why does the FDA and the AMA harass and inhibit those who market oils, herbs, and natural supplements that help heal people, keep them well, and exemplify the tradition of Hippocrates to "First, do no harm?" At the same time, why do they endorse, finance, and encourage those who market pharmaceuticals that harm more than they heal and which make us sick—even to death?

Witchcraft and the Roots of Medicine

The U.S. Government figures quoted in the previous paragraphs mean that the ordained guardians of our health kill twice as many people every week as died in the September 11, 2001, terrorist attacks on the New York World Trade Center and Pentagon. But the news media won't report the scandal of deaths from legal drugs because their incomes are so greatly dependent on advertising revenues from pharmaceutical companies.

Rev. Jim Lynn, in his book, *The Miracle of Healing in your Church Today,* says it bluntly: "Medicine that heals is of God. Medicine that harms is of evil." In other words, "Medicine that harms is of Satan."

Modern medicine has been largely reduced to the administration of drugs, all of which have undesirable side effects, sometimes fatal. The roots of atheistic medicine are revealed in the roots of the word, "pharmaceutical." It comes from the Greek word, "pharmakeuein," meaning "to practice witchcraft," and the word "pharmokon," meaning "poison." In Revelations 9:21; 18:23; 21:8; and 22:15 we find four references to sorcerers or sorcery all of which have been translated from the Greek pharmakeia, pharmakeus, or pharmakos.

Furthermore, in Galatians 5:19-21, Paul lists the "acts of the flesh" (KJV, NRSV) or the "acts of the sinful nature" (NIV) as "adultery, fornication, uncleanness, lasciviousness, idolatry, witchcraft, hatred, etc. . ." The Greek word for idolatry here is "eidololatreia" which means "worship of that which is not God." The English word, "idolatry," comes from this Greek root, whose dictionary definition is "excessive attachment or trust in a person or thing." These phrases could well describe the attachment and excessive trust that many have for their doctors and/or the medical system in general? The Greek word, eidololatreia, is found also in I Corinthians 10:14, Colossians 3:5, and I Peter 4-3 where, in every instance, we are advised by scripture to avoid it.

Now consider the term, "witchcraft," which Paul lists right after idolatry in these verses. Most interpret this to mean such things as hexes, incantations, voodoo, ouija boards, spells, seances, satanic rituals, divination, consulting with familiar spirits, necromancy, and things like that. In the *Old Testament*, the Hebrew words translated into English as "witchcraft" or "witch" do imply exactly those things. The corresponding Hebrew words are "kashaph" or "keshaphim." But in the *New Testament*, the word translated as "witchcraft" has quite a different meaning and does not refer to the practices listed above. The Greek word used here by Paul is "pharmakeia" which means "medicine or drug from a pharmacy."

The *Bible* seems to be advising us to avoid such medicines, yet many church-going Americans spend more for drugs from a pharmacy, prescribed by a doctor in whose hands they trust their very lives, than they do for food or for charitable causes, including contributions to their own church. The satanic roots of the pharmaceutical industry become even more evident when one understands the ways that man-made drugs work.

How the Human Body Works

In the last chapter we discussed how your body is a system of 100 trillion cells. Consider these as 100 trillion employees whose job it is to run the corporation of your body smoothly and in good health. Most of the time they do a pretty good job, which is a miracle in and of itself. Any employer or manager who has had to direct the activities of even a small number of employees knows what a challenge it is to keep things running smoothly and productively on a daily basis. Yet, our beautifully organized bodies do that with little or no conscious effort on our parts. That is because God is the head of the corporation and has imbued every cell with intelligence—six gigabytes worth for every cell.

The way these 100 trillion cells act cooperatively and in harmony is by continuous intracellular communication. Cells and body systems communicate between each other in two ways: (1) by electricity through the neurons (This is your email system) and (2) by hormones, peptides, neurotransmitters, steroids, and other molecules (known as "ligands") that travel between cells and systems to carry messages (This is your FedEx® courier system). The first means of communication is by the nervous system (electrical). The second means is by the endocrine system (chemical).

When your body requires a fast response, it sends an instantaneous email. For example, if your hand comes in contact with something hot, your reflexes fire an email directly to the muscles to say "Move it quick! Your hand is burning!"

When your body is in need of an activity that is complex or must be sustained for a period of time, it sends couriers to pass the instructions to the cells. Hence, when your body needs insulin to process sugar, hormones pass from the brain to the liver to the pancreas and back to the liver, explaining the process to the DNA intelligence of all the necessary cells to carry out the desired function.

The portals into the cell's memory are called "receptor sites." Each one of your 100 trillion cells has tens of thousands of receptor sites. Each receptor site has specific functions and a lock that requires a specific key. For a hormone or other information carrying molecule to pass its information to a cell, it has to hold the right key. That is why a specific hormone can circulate throughout your body and affect only the cells for which its key was designed to fit.

Your body makes thousands of hormones millions of times every day to carry out the complex task of keeping every body cell and system informed as to its task at the moment as well as briefing cells on what their neighbors are doing at any given moment. By this incredible system of intracellular communication, devised by God, the master engineer, our 100 trillion cells work in harmony and we stay healthy and vigorous for his service.

How Pharmaceuticals Work

Pharmaceuticals are specifically designed to block specific receptor sites or to pass false information to certain cells in order to trick the body into giving up symptoms. Thus, if you have an ache or a pain or a runny nose or high blood pressure or any other symptom, prescription drugs are designed to find the cells that give rise to those symptoms and trick them into stopping. For example, antihistamines are drugs designed to block the histamine receptors so that we won't sneeze and cough and produce the unpleasant mucous that comes with some viral infections. Opposing symptoms is what allopathic medicine is all about and is what the word "allopath" means.

But symptoms are messengers to get our attention that a problem exists so we can deal with it. Allopaths mistake the messenger for the problem. Instead of trying to interpret the message and address the root of the problem, they kill the messenger.

Hence, when doctors prescribe symptom-relieving drugs, your problem may appear to have disappeared, but it hasn't. You have simply forced the body to produce another set of symptoms (usually more severe) at some later time to try to get your attention to deal with the real problem which is still there. Hence, one may start with a simple illness that over a period of time gradually escalates into a serious chronic debilitating disease like multiple sclerosis or cancer.

When people take more than one prescription drug, inevitably there will be adverse inter-reactions between the drugs. Why is this so? Because drugs are telling lies to your body. You can tell one lie and, perhaps, get by. But when you tell one lie after another, contradictions eventually occur and the whole system of lies collapses. And who is the father of lies? "The devil," says the scriptures. "He is a liar, and the father of it." (John 8:44) "Satan deceives the whole world," says John in Revelation 12:9.

In I Corinthians 14:33 we read that "God is not the author of confusion." Prescription drugs are a major cause of serious illness because they confuse the body's 100 trillion cells so they cannot work in harmony and health any longer. As a result, prescription drugs have become the third leading cause of death in the United States, exceeded only by heart disease and cancer. Medicines that kill and confuse cannot be of God. (See Rev. Lynn's book, *The Miracle of Healing in Your Church Today*, for more on this.)

Essential Oils vs. Drugs

By contrast to pharmaceuticals, God's medicine in the form of essential oils works in a different way.

As described in the previous chapter, essential oils

contain: (1) Phenylpropanoids that cleanse receptor sites, (2) Sesquiterpenes that erase incorrect information in the cellular memory, and (3) Monoterpenes that restore God's original information into the DNA.

In simple terms, what oils do is to stimulate the body to return to normality. They do this by telling truths to your cells. Since oils all work toward the same end, the restoration of normal, healthy bodily function as originally intended by God the maker, they all work in harmony.

Hence, unlike drugs that lie and contradict one another eventually creating confusion, chaos and disease in the body, oils agree with each other in their overall objectives, work in harmony, and move the body toward a state of health.

This is why you can apply many oils on your body at once and not have an adverse inter-reaction because when everyone is telling the truth, there can be no contradictions. By contrast, even a small number of lies is likely to result in contradictions which is why even a few drugs taken together will produce undesirable consequences.

In Hebrews 6:18 we read, "It is impossible for God to lie." Therefore, the essential oils he created for us as medicines and promoters of well-being are full of truth. As John says in his Gospel, "Ye shall know the truth and the truth shall make ye free." (John 8:32)

Now you know the difference between man-made pharmaceuticals and God-made oils: The former are packs of lies while the latter are bearers of truth.

Sometimes a Deception is Necessary

I am not saying there is no place for pharmaceuticals. Sometimes we don't quite tell the truth to children because they aren't ready to receive it. Those sorts of deceptions are considered necessary to protect the immature child until they can receive the full truth.

There are also times when deceiving the body to trick it into giving up a symptom is life-saving. But sooner or later, the body needs the truth. The value of a pharmaceutical is for temporary relief, which is sometimes necessary in order to survive until the real problem can be effectively addressed.

It seems that in an emergency, drugs can be okay so long as their use is temporary. Habitual use is not good and never leads to true healing, health or wholeness. As for cures and permanent healing, allopathic medicine has few answers. Drugs are never the answer for overcoming chronic illness. You need to look elsewhere.

Some may argue that when a surgeon removes a diseased portion of your body, like a cancerous breast, that you are healed from cancer in that body part for as long as you live. But such extreme measures are not "healing." You have been maimed for life. You will never be complete again. Healing is when you are made whole and well, restored to the perfection that God originally intended for us as his creations. To be healed of breast cancer is to remain intact and fully restored to health and wellness.

The allopathic model does not understand the concept of healing because healing is a spiritual event, not a medical one. There is only one source of healing and that is God. The best a physician can do is to be a vessel, a vehicle, and a facilitator. This takes humility, surrender, and attunement with God. These attributes are neither taught nor encouraged in medical school.

What the Bible Says About Doctors

The *Bible* doesn't have much to say about physicians. They were present, but the major responsibilities for diagnosing and prescribing therapeutic regimens among the Jews was delegated to the priesthood while childbirth and the care of women were mostly in the hands of midwives. (Exodus 1:15-21)

The word, "doctor," only occurs three times in the *Bible* (Luke 2:46; 5:17; and Acts 5:34). The author of the verses containing the word, in all cases, was Luke, who was, himself, a physician. Luke wrote the Gospel bearing his name as well as the Acts of the Apostles. In all three cases the references are to rabbis, teachers, or "doctors of the law." The word "doctor," in the *Bible*, is never used to indicate a healer or a practitioner of the medical arts. It means "teacher."

The word "physician," used in the sense of a healer or administrator of oils and medicines, is found eleven times in the *Bible*, but not always in a sense that is very flattering or commendable.

The first Biblical reference to a physician is in the last chapter of Genesis (50:2) where Joseph ordered the Egyptian physicians to embalm his father, Israel, which they did using essential oils of cedarwood, frankincense, myrrh, and others. In this case, the assignment of the physicians was not to heal, but to administer oils, herbs, minerals, and spices to preserve a corpse.

The Case of the Faithless King

The second Biblical reference to physicians has to do with King Asa in II Chronicles 16:11-14. It seems that Asa contracted a disease in his feet that got worse and worse. According to the *Bible*, he did not seek the help of the Lord in his infirmity, but instead sought the aid of physicians. As a result—he died.

There is an important lesson in this story, applicable

to us today. When afflicted with disease, many request to be on prayer lists and seek God's aid with their lips, but in their hearts their faith is in doctors and hospitals. Just like the story of Asa, they often die as a result—having misplaced their faith in a secular source when the sole source of healing is God.

During King Asa's burial ceremonies, he was laid on a bed "filled with sweet odors and various kinds of spices prepared by the apothecaries' art: and they made a very great fire in his honor." (II Chronicles 16:14) The burning would have included highly combustible essential oils which, upon ignition, made a great and spectacular fire. Such a burning would also act like a giant source of incense, filling the city with a great cloud of aromatic smoke. According to the *Bible*, the King was then "buried in the tomb that he had hewn out for himself in the city of David."

Job Refuses Secular Medicine and Lives

When Job was smitten with aches and pains and boils all over his body, his suffering was so intense that he wished for death to relieve him. But his faith in God remained unabated. When his worldly friends came to offer uninvited advice on the cause and cure of his ills, he listened patiently for a while and then launched into a long reproof.

Acknowledging the omnipotence of God (Job 12), he then vehemently accuses his friends of being "forgers of lies and physicians of no value." (Job 13:4). Then he states his famous and ultimate affirmation of faith in God, "Though he slay me, yet will I trust in Him: I will maintain mine own ways before Him. He also shall be my salvation." (Job 13:15-16)

While Job's friends proposed secular solutions to his trials, he remained steadfast in his conviction that God would be his redeemer and would be sufficient to save him. Refusing all worldly advice, he prayed, waited upon the Lord, saw him with his own eyes (Job 42:12), was healed completely, and lived to the ripe old age of 140. (Job 42:16)

The Woman Who Bled for Twelve Years

A rather uncomplimentary story of the physicians of Jesus' times is told in Mark 5:25-34 and Luke 8:43-48. The story is about a sick woman who gave all of her money to doctors and and yet continued to get sicker and sicker—an example that matches the experiences of many people today.

According to Mark: "A certain woman which had an issue of blood twelve years, and had suffered many things of many physicians, and had spent all that she had, and was nothing bettered, but rather grew worse, when she had heard of Jesus, came in the crowd behind, and touched his garment. For she said, if I may touch but his clothes, I shall be whole."

Matthew and John don't relate this incident, but it is interesting that Luke, a physician himself, also tells this unflattering story, saying "she had spent all she had on physicians, yet no one could cure her."

Luke was, evidently, a different kind of physician than were his colleagues in that day. He was a follower of Jesus and a man of prayer. In Paul's letter to the Colossians, he refers to his physician friend as "Luke, the beloved physician." (Colossians 4:14) It is physicians like Luke that Christians should seek out today—healers who pray and acknowledge God as the source of all healing, physicians who are not atheistic in their practice.

Did Biblical Priests Know Reflexology?

The role of the priesthood in diagnosing, prescribing, and administering oils is partially described in Leviticus 13-14. There is a cleansing ceremony for leprosy the

priests were to perform on the person and a parallel ritual to be performed on the house in which the leper
lived. Both rituals involved cedarwood and hyssop and
a "log of oil" which would have been beaten olive oil containing aromatics. A log is a unit of volume equal to
about 10 fluid ounces, or 2/3 of a pint. (Leviticus 14: 6,
10-12, 24, 49, 52)

During the ritual, the priest is to take some oil and
anoint the top of the leper's right ear, the right thumb,
and the right big toe. (Leviticus 14:17) The choices of
these reflex points and these oils is very interesting in
light of today's understanding of reflexology.

The upper portion of the ear is the trigger point for
releasing emotional issues regarding the mother and
father. The thumb is where fears of the unknown and
mental blocks to acquiring wisdom can be released. The
big toe is another point for clearing addictions or compulsive behavior. The scent of hyssop is a releaser of
swallowed emotions and a spiritual cleanser of past sin,
immorality, and evil spirits. Cedarwood oil can clear
emotions of many kinds, but is particularly suited to
deal with conceit and pride.

Could it be that the ancient Levites understood the
underlying emotional basis of degenerative diseases like
leprosy? Could it be that they also understood the emotionally releasing powers of essential oils and the emotional release points of the body as well?

Jesus and the Ten Lepers

The medical authority of the priests was also recognized by Jesus in a story told by Luke. It seems that
there were ten Samaritan lepers who approached Jesus
asking to be healed. Jesus' response was, "Go show
yourselves to the priests." As they headed to the temple,
they discovered themselves to be healed.

The reason Jesus directed them to the priests is

because only a priest had the authority to diagnose leprosy or to pronounce a person healed and free of the disease. Hence, in the eyes of the Jews of that day, Jesus needed the authentification of a priest's examination to verify the actuality of his miraculous healing. (Luke 17:12-19)

This is not unlike some spiritual healers of today who may seek the diagnosis of licensed physicians before and after their healings so that their results will be accepted and believed.

There is no denying that physical healing was a major part of Jesus' ministry and teaching. He trained his disciples also to be healers and the tradition was carried on for many decades, if not centuries, in the early church. During the first few centuries of Christianity, there were even reports of several raisings from the dead. (See Lynn's book, *Miracle of Healing in Your Church Today*.)

Separation of Church and State

The foregoing discussion is not meant to imply that modern allopathic medicine is all wrong. We are pointing out the fact that modern health care can be very destructive to people's lives—physically, emotionally, spiritually, and financially. We believe the root of this problem lies in the atheistic basis for current practice. What we are saying is that the application of any healing art without prayer and acknowledgement of God as the healer is likely to cause more harm than good, facilitating sickness instead of health.

The political idea of separation of church and state is a good thing when it comes to protecting our freedoms to worship and exercise our religious convictions. But separation of God from medicine is a deadly mistake. The statistics quoted earlier in this chapter prove that. The data given here is only a tiny sample of the dangers of modern medicine. There are whole books that detail these hazards in every field, from psychiatry, to oncology, to cardiology, to obstetrics and gynecology.

Despite their difficiencies, dangers, and deceits, there is a time for seeking the help of the medical system. There are times when their services can be of benefit and can save lives. Only prayer and God's guidance can enable you to make the right choices in this regard at those times.

A Scriptural Tribute to Physicians

The *Bible* has few words to say regarding physicians, and, as stated earlier, not all of them are very kind. However, the Catholic *Bible*, as well as the original Protestant *King James Version* of 1611, includes the fifteen books of the *Old Testament Apocrypha* as scripture. Among the Apocryphal books is one called Sirach (also known as Ecclesiasticus) written between 195 B.C. and 171 B.C. Sirach has a tribute to the ideal, God-fearing physician as follows:

> "Honor the physician with the honor due him, according to your need of him, for the Lord created him; for healing comes from the Most High. . . The Lord created medicines from the earth, and a sensible man will not despise them. . . God gave skill to men that he might be glorified in his marvelous works. By them he heals and takes away pain. . . My son, when you are sick do not be negligent, but pray to the Lord, and he will heal you. Give up your faults and direct your hands aright, and cleanse your heart from all sin. . . There is a time when success lies in the hands of physicians, for they too will pray to the Lord that he should grant them success in diagnosis and in healing, for the sake of preserving life. (Sirach 38:1-14)

This passage is an excellent summary of the proper role of physicians as instruments of God. It is a good description of the ideal patient as a participant in their healing and the receiver of grace. It also describes the relationships between prayer, sin, repentance, healing, and God—the source of all healing and the creator of natural medicines.

Who are the Real Priests?

The anointing oil of Exodus 30:23-25, containing healing oils of myrrh, cinnamon, calamus, cassia, and olive was, for a long time, restricted in its use to the priesthood and to the anointing of kings by the prophets. But who are the real priests of God? According to Peter, we are all "a chosen race, a royal priesthood, a holy nation, God's own people..." (I Peter 2:9). In Luke we read that Jesus appointed his followers (not just his chosen twelve) and sent them "to heal the sick." (Luke 10:1-9) We are all called and authorized to anoint and heal.

The priests of the *Bible* had a long list of duties, most of which are described throughout Leviticus as well as I Chronicles 9:26-30. They were to be the leaders of all activities concerning worship—including offerings, sacrifices, and prayers. They were to serve as spiritual counselors and hearers of confession. They were judges, lawyers, and enforcers of ecclesiastic law—determining guilts and executing punishments. They were the keepers of the perpetual fire that burned night and day on the altar of the temple as a symbol of undying devotion to God. (Leviticus 6:12-13; 24:2-4) They were responsible for certain medical diagnoses and treatments. They were the apothecaries and perfumers who mixed the various oils and herbs for anointing, for incense, and for healing. (I Chronicles 9:30) They also cared for the temple buildings and grounds, keeping them clean, attractive, and in good repair. In addition to all of that, they were expected to live exemplary lives of righteousness. Hence, they were to be pastors, counselors, judges, physicians, medicine makers, maintenance engineers, and models of righteous living—all in one.

So how does that relate to us today? We answer that with a series of questions:

• What is the ultimate temple in which we all must worship?

• Whose duty is it to keep it clean, attractive, and in good condition?

• And who is the priest of your temple who must conduct the worship, keep the altar flames burning, assess illnesses as they arise, decide on the best courses to take in addressing a medical problem, and be a good example of living a spiritual and clean life?

The *Bible* answers these questions clearly in several places:

"Behold, the kingdom of God is within you."   (Luke 17:21)

"Ye are the temple of the living God."   (II Corinthians 6:16)

"Know not that ye are the temple of God and that the spirit of God dwelleth within you?"   (I Corinthians 3:16)

"What? Know ye not that your body is the temple of the Holy Ghost which is in you, which ye have of God." (I Corinthians 6:19)

"Like living stones, let yourselves be built into a spiritual house, to be a holy priesthood, to offer spiritual sacrifices acceptable to God through Jesus Christ."   (I Peter 2:5)

Everyone is a High Priest of Their Own Temple

The primary and most important temple in which each of us must worship and find God is the temple of our own body. It is in that temple, and no other, that we must ultimately seek and find Him.

• And who must care for that temple? We must.

• Who must ultimately carry out the worship, offerings, sacrifices, and prayers in establishing a personal relationship with God? We must.

• Who is responsible for keeping the flame of love for God alive on the altar of our hearts? We are.

• Who is responsible for keeping our consciences clear and our moral behavior free from transgression as examples of a child of God? We are.

• Who must be the one to initiate the process of repentance and correction of lifestyles when we err? We must.

• Who must be the first to take responsibility for the diagnosing and treatment of any illness in our bodily temples? We must.

• And who must ultimately be the one to choose our medicines and remedies to keep our temples sound, vigorous, and in good repair? We must.

It all boils down to embracing individual, personal responsibility and surrendering to God in the faith that he will help us in all things and circumstances.

Therefore, in the ultimate sense, when we stand alone before God, it is incumbent upon each and every one of us to accept the duties of the priests that we are. It is we who must conduct our own worship within our own personal temples to find God and receive his peace, his love, his wisdom, and his guidance. It is we who must take responsibility for maintaining our temples in good healthy condition so that they may serve both us and God to the best of their capabilities.

Therefore, we are all entitled to use anointing oils on ourselves and to administer them to others. We are all ordained and appointed by God for this. We are all anointed as priests and sent by Christ to heal. We are all endowed, not only with the spiritual and temporal duties of the priesthood, but also the healing responsibilities for the maintenance of our own wellness by right living and right thinking and with authority to pass this on to others. (I Peter 2:5,9; Luke 10:1-11)

> "And they went out and preached that men should repent. And they cast out many devils, and anointed with oil many that were sick, and healed them." (Mark 6:11-13)

> "Is any sick among you, let him call for the elders of the church; let them pray over him, anointing him with oil in the name of the Lord." (James 5:14)

> "Beloved, I wish above all things that you may prosper and be in health, even as your soul prospers." (III John 2)

Chapter Four

The Biblical Meaning of Anointment

The most common Biblical act we associate with oil is anointing—which is mentioned 156 times. Almost everyone raised in a Judeo-Christian society has memorized, or is at least familiar with, the Twenty-Third Psalm. One of its most familiar lines is, "Thou anointest my head with oil." Since that line was written by a king, and the anointer was no less than God, himself, the oil of this verse could well have been the "holy anointing oil" of the Israelites, which was a blend that was 82% essential oils (myrrh, cassia, cinnamon, and calamus) in a base oil of olive. (Exodus 30:23-24) In any event, we know that the oil to which David was referring was fragrant because anointing oils always contained at least some aromatic ingredients, if not 100%.

The true and ancient meaning of "anoint" has been lost in modern times. It has almost been forgotten and has not been widely practiced for centuries. Many Christian ministers use oils for healing services from time to time, but they usually apply only trace amounts—a dab on the forehead or a little on the crown. They usually consider the oil as symbolic, only, and do not recognize any innate medicinal value to be contained in the oils themselves. As a matter of convenience and cost, some ministers even use grocery store oils such as Wesson® and Mazola®. These anointings may have ritual value as ceremonies of consecration, but they are not really Biblical when it comes to anointment for healing.

Lots of Oil and Always Essential

In Psalms 133:2 the writer describes the anointing of Aaron with "precious ointment upon the head, that ran down upon the beard, even Aaron's beard: that went down to the skirts of his garments," (KJV) or "like the precious oil on the head, running down the beard, upon the beard of Aaron, running down over the collar of his robes." (NRSV)

This is no small amount of oil. Neither was it pure olive oil since the Biblical adjective "precious" was never applied to olive oil alone, but always indicated the use of essential oils such as cassia, hyssop, frankincense, spikenard, galbanum, myrrh, onycha, cinnamon, and/or calamus. In Biblical times essential oils were often mixed in a vegetable oil base such as olive, flaxseed, walnut, sesame, or almond. But vegetable oils, alone, were never used for anointings. In fact, the word "anointment" is literally "an ointment." Biblical ointments were always composed of essential oils.

In the *New Testament* we read of "precious ointment" or "oil" literally being poured over Jesus on two occasions during Holy Week in his final sojourn to Jerusalem before his arrest. (Matthew 26:7, 12; Mark 14:3; John 12:3-8). Here, again, we find copious amounts of oil being used—oil that was costly and in this case, consisted entirely of essential oils of spikenard and myrrh. (See Chapter 10 on Myrrh.)

Jesus also schooled his disciples in the spiritual art of anointing to bring about healing using oil (usually olive) that contained precious spices and other aromatic oils. (Mark 6:13) A fuller discussion of this is given at the end of this chapter.

Pour it On

The idea of pouring an anointing oil on the head is mentioned in the *Bible* several times.

"Thou shalt take the anointing oil and pour it upon his head and anoint him." (Exodus 29:7)

"And Moses took the anointing oil. . . and he poured of the anointing oil upon Aaron's head and anointed him to sanctify him." (Leviticus 8:10-12)

"And he that was the high priest among his brethren, upon whose head the anointing oil was poured. . ." (Leviticus 21:10)

"Then Samuel took a vial of oil and poured it upon (Saul's) head and kissed him and said, is it not because the Lord hath anointed thee to be captain over his inheritance?" (I Samuel 10:1)

"Then take the box of oil and pour it on (Jehu's) head and say, thus saith the Lord, I have anointed thee king over Israel." (I Kings 9:3)

"And he arose and went into the house (of Jehu) and he poured the oil on his head, and said unto him, thus saith the Lord God of Israel, I have anointed thee king over the people of the Lord, even over Israel." (II Kings 9:6)

Now please don't read these scriptures and go out and pour a whole bottle of cypress, hyssop, frankincense, or some other pure essential oil on your head or somebody else's head. Some of the oils referred to above were probably pure essential oils and some were mixtures of fatty carrier oils and aromatic oils. One must use discretion and common sense. Some essential oils, while safe to apply neat in small quantities, are too strong to apply undiluted in large quantities.

The Biblical Meaning of Anoint

According to *Harper's Bible Dictionary*, the *Interpreter's Dictionary of the Bible*, and *Young's*

Analytic Concordance, the words translated from the Hebrew and Greek as "anoint" meant "to cover, rub, or smear the head or body (or object) with oil" and, in some cases, the word meant "to pour oil over the head or body (or object)." A commonly used Hebrew word for anoint was "masach" or "mishcah" or "moshchah." It is interesting that these Hebrew variations of the word for anoint are similar to the English word "massage" both in meaning and in pronunciation.

It is clear that a true Biblical anointing was not a small dot of vegetable oil applied with a light touch of a finger or with the simple laying on of hands. A true anointing was usually more than that. It often involved a considerable amount of oil, usually consisting of a carrier, such as olive, containing aromatic oils or consisting of essential oils by themselves. Sometimes there was some rubbing and smearing of the oils to various parts of the body. As an example, consider the women who anointed Jesus feet. (Luke 7:36-50; John 12:1-8) They apparently massaged his feet with the oil and kissed them as well.

Raindrop technique is a modern-day massage protocol of applying oils for healing and wellness. Seven single oils and three blends are used. The procedure takes about an hour. With the right attitudes on the parts of giver and receiver, raindrop can be considered as an anointing in the Biblical sense of the word. (See page 325 with info on *The Raindrop Study*.)

The Hebrew term, "masach," is also the root of the term "Messiah." Since the *New Testament* was not in Hebrew, but in Greek, the Hebrew word "Messiah" appears only twice in the KJV (John 1:41 and 4:25) but the Greek term "Kristos," or "Christ," appears 361 times. Kristos literally means "the anointed one."

Variations on the Word: "Anoint"

The word "anoint" and its derivatives occurs 156 times in the *Bible*, but use of the word does not always connote the use of oils. In John 9:6, a blind man is "anointed" with a little piece of clay that Jesus moistened with his spit. When the blind man began to see, his friends inquired, "How were thine eyes opened?" To this he replied, "A man named Jesus made clay and anointed my eyes." (John 9:11) In this case, the anointment was with mud, not oil.

Another use of the word "anoint" is in the sense of being appointed or chosen by God or the Holy Spirit. This is an anointment that requires no oil. It is an anointment of spirit. This sense of the word is used ten times in the *Bible* and is found in Psalms 2:2; Lamentations 4:20; Ezekiel 28:14; Habakkuk 3:13; Zechariah 4:14; Luke 4:18; Acts 4:27; 10:38; II Corinthians 1:21; and I John 2:27.

Any time a priest was anointed, it always implied the use of the aromatic holy anointing oil of Exodus 30:23-24. Incidents of priests being anointed are found more than 30 times in the *Bible*. And as for kings, they were always anointed with fragrant oils of some kind. There are 61 royal anointings in the *Bible* and essential oils would have been involved in every instance.

Anointing as an Act of Hospitality

The term anoint was also used for an act of hospitality practiced among the Jews. When notable guests came to visit, as a welcome and a greeting, a little perfumed oil was poured on the head and feet and massaged into the skin. For a weary traveler who had come many miles on foot in a pair of open sandals or, perhaps, even barefoot, such an experience would be relaxing and pleasant, indeed.

Plain vegetable oil was never applied alone. The massage oil, even if it was mostly olive, almond, or some other fatty oil, would always contain fragrant oils as well.

In addition to the pleasant experience of the massage for the guest, the aromatic ingredients of the oil also had the practical benefit of a deodorant. Since offering your road-weary visitor an opportunity to shower and freshen up was not an option available in Biblical times, and since sweat and body odor were a normal state of the body in those days, anointment with a fragrant oil was wonderful thing for both the receiver and the giver. (see Luke 7:46)

Another thing that essential oils did for the feet was to soothe any cuts or abrasions that might have occurred during the travel and assist in their healing. Essential oils are not only antiseptic in preventing infections, they are also analgesic in reducing pain so that one's "aching" feet would receive instant relief.

Anointing Things Instead of People

People are not the only things anointed with oil in the *Bible*. In Genesis 31:31 there is mention of a stone pillar that was anointed to seal a covenant between God and Jacob.

In II Samuel 1:21 and Isaiah 21:5, shields are anointed to strengthen and sanctify them for God's protection in battle.

In Exodus 29:2, Leviticus 2:4; 7:12, and Numbers 6:15, it was wafers of unleavened bread that were anointed, which were then eaten. The anointing oil for the bread would have been either frankincense or the holy anointing oil of myrrh, cassia, cinnamon, calamus, and olive. In this way, some essential oils were taken internally.

In Exodus 30:26-29; 40:9-11, Leviticus 8:10-11, and Numbers 7:1, Moses anoints the tabernacle and all that was inside to sanctify them. This included the Ark of the Covenant, the various altars, and all their "vessels" which included candlesticks, bowls, goblets, knives, flasks, pots, and alabaster boxes that contained precious ointments. Some of these could have been made of wood or pottery, but in a temple or tabernacle they were more likely to be made of gold, silver, bronze or copper. Moses also anoints the "laver," which was a large copper or bronze bowl containing the water used daily by the priests for cleansing themselves in preparation for their religious duties.

The oil that Moses used for this was the holy oil whose formula is given in Exodus 30:23-24—which, being high in phenylpropanoids, would have been an excellent disinfectant, protecting the priests from the spread of disease by their shared use of the laver and the handling of many animals on a daily basis.

The Holy Anointing Oil of Moses

All of the oils used for anointing in the *Bible* contained aromatic components. Although olive oil was commonly used, it was never used by itself but mixed with aromatic oils. In Exodus 30:23-24 God gives a recipe to Moses for a "holy anointing oil" as follows:

Myrrh	500 shekels
Cassia	500 shekels
Cinnamon	250 shekels
Calamus	250 shekels
Olive oil	1 hin

A shekel was about 12 grams in weight, or approximately 15 milliliters, or 0.5 fluid ounces in volume. A hin was about half a liter or half a quart or 16 fluid ounces in volume. Converting the above into consistent modern units we get the following:

Myrrh	25 fl.oz. = 3 cups	27%
Cassia	25 fl.oz. = 3 cups	27%
Cinnamon	12 fl.oz. = 1.5 cups	14%
Calamus	12 fl.oz. = 1.5 cups	14%
Olive oil	16 fl.oz. = 2 cups	18%

These quantities and proportions would yield eleven cups, or 2.75 quarts of holy anointing oil. As you can see, the result would be 82% essential oil and 18% carrier. For a small quantity you can change ounces into drops (i.e. 25 drops myrrh, 12 drops cinnamon, 16 drops olive, etc.) which would yield about 4 ml or 1/8 fl. oz. of anointing oil. There are approximately 600 drops of oil in one fluid ounce. A 15 ml bottle oil is 0.5 ounces and contains about 300 drops.

It should also be noted here that the olive oil to be used is specified by scripture to be the "first" or "beaten" oil of olive. (Exodus 27:20; 29:40; Leviticus 24:2; Numbers 28:5) In modern language, this means "virgin" or "extra virgin" olive oils which are aromatic and not the second non-aromatic grades that are labeled as "refined" or "pure." There are also "light" or "medium" grades of olive oil, but these are second grade with a bit of virgin oil mixed in for a touch of flavor. For more on this, read the chapter entitled "Olive: The Other Healing Oil of the *Bible*."

Responsibility for mixing and maintaining a supply of this holy blend in *Old Testament* times fell to the priestly caste—the Levites, the descendants of Aaron. In that capacity they were referred to as "apothecaries," or "perfumers." (I Chronicles 9:30)

Following God's recipe for the oil given to Moses, the Lord issued the following instructions:

"And thou shalt make it an oil of holy ointment, an ointment compound after the art of the apothecary: it shall be an holy anointing oil. And thou shalt anoint the tabernacle and the congregation therewith, and the ark of the testimony, and the table and all his vessels, and the candlestick and his vessels, and the altar of incense. And the altar of burnt offering with all his vessels, and the laver and his foot. And thou shalt sanctify them, that they may be most holy: whatsoever toucheth them shall be holy. And thou shalt anoint Aaron and his sons, and consecrate them, that they may minister unto me in the priest's office. And thou shalt speak unto the children of Israel, saying, This shall be an holy anointing oil unto me throughout your generations." (Exodus 30:25-31)

Holy Incense

After the recipe for holy anointing oil, God then gave Moses a formula for incense as follows:

"Take unto thee sweet spices, stacte, and onycha, and galbanum; these sweet spices with pure frankincense: of each shall there be a like weight. And thou shalt make it a perfume, a confection after the art of the apothecary, tempered together, pure and holy." (Exodus 30:34-35)

Stacte is another word for myrrh. Myrrh is the only ingredient that was a part of both the holy anointing oil and the holy incense. Other incenses were used by the Israelites employing the oils of spikenard, cassia, saffron, costus, mace, and sweet flag. Some of these others were, perhaps, burned in temples as well as homes and businesses. But only the formula given above was designated as "holy," delivered by God, himself.

The fact that myrrh is found in both the incense and the anointing oil formulated by God may have to do with the fact that myrrh is one of the most effective fixing oils of all time and one of the most used. A fixative is an oil that, when mixed with other aromatic oils, causes their fragrances to last longer. This is knowledge that would normally only be possessed by professional perfumers or aromatherapists. The designating of myrrh by God as an ingredient in both of these holy preparations is further evidence that He was the first and original aromatherapist.

Myrrh, in fact, is the most mentioned oil of the scriptures and was used as a fixative in many ointments. (See Chapter Ten)

Smoking as a Form of Aromatherapy

When oils are used as incense, some of their therapeutic value is lost in the burning, but not all of it by any means. If this were so, the nicotine of tobacco cigarettes, the cannabis of marijuana, and the morphine of opium would all be destroyed before it could be inhaled. Breathing smoke is, in fact, a very effective way to absorb the active ingredients of a plant. Anyone who has had the misfortune of inhaling or walking through the smoke of a pile of burning weeds containing poison ivy vines will know that the allergenic oil of poison ivy is still potent and painfully dangerous in that form.

The potency of aromatic smoke was a fact well understood by the peoples of Biblical times. In fact, fumigation (releasing aromatic molecules into the air by smoke) was a common way of administering the healing powers of essential oils in Biblical times. In Numbers 16:46-50 Aaron stops a plague among the Israelites by fumigating their encampment with vapors of frankincense, galbanum, onycha, and myrrh.

Today we recommend diffusing the oils at room temperature or rubbing (anointing) them directly on the body as a more efficient and cost-effective way to derive their benefits.

Holy Things for Holy Purposes

The verses in Exodus that follow the formulas for holy anointing oil and holy incense are a caveat against using holy substances for secular purposes:

> "Upon man's flesh shall it (the oil) not be poured, neither shall ye make any other like it, after the composition of it: it is holy, and it shall be holy unto you. Whosoever compoundeth any like it, or whosoever putteth any of it upon a stranger, shall even be cut off from his people." (Exodus 30:32-33)

> "And as for the perfume (holy incense) which thou shalt make, ye shall not make to yourselves according to the composition thereof: it shall be unto thee holy for the Lord. Whosoever shall make like unto that, to smell thereto, shall even be cut off from his people." (Exodus 30:37-38)

If you were thinking of mixing up a batch of the holy anointing oil to try yourself or of making some holy incense to burn in your home and are concerned about the warnings against doing so in Exodus, then don't do it. However, according to some interpretations of the scriptures, these prohibitions are no longer in effect—cancelled by God himself as stated in Jeremiah 3:8.

From the Old Covenant to the New

These formulas, given by God to Moses, were part of the original covenant between the Lord and the Israelites established through Abraham in the fifteenth chapter of Genesis and reaffirmed to Moses in Exodus, Chapters 19-24. By this covenant the children of Israel were to be God's chosen people to be specially blessed—but there were conditions. The Israelites were to obey certain laws and rules. If they did not keep their side of the promise, then the covenant could be retracted by God.

The conditions of the first covenant consist basically of following the Ten Commandments (Exodus 20:1-17). But Israel did not keep God's commandments, breaking them repeatedly over many decades. Finally, in Jeremiah 3:8 God delivers a bill of divorcement that nullifies the covenant. Jeremiah 31:31-34 then proposes a future new covenant that would not be conditional on external conformity with the law, but on the internal conditions of one's heart and the sincerity of one's soul. The new covenant would be based on individuals actually "knowing God."

To Christians, that new covenant was initiated with the death and resurrection of Christ. According to the writer of Hebrews, the New Covenant is unconditional, based on the eternal unchanging love of God and Christ and not on the fickle behavior of people. (Hebrews 7:22; 8:8-13; 9:15; 12:24)

The point is this. According to some authorities, the prohibition against using the formulas for holy anointing oil and holy incense in Exodus 30 were part of the old covenant which is no longer in effect. However, not all authorities agree on this. It is a matter you will have to decide for yourself.

Applying Oils for Healing & Wellness

The ingredients to the holy oil and incense are not all easily obtainable. It is particularly difficult to obtain the oils of calamus and onycha. However, there is one blend commercially available called Exodus II™. While not a duplicate of Moses' formulas, it does contain the oils of the Exodus formulas (except for onycha) with the addition of hyssop and spikenard. Exodus II™ contains the following oils:

Cassia, Hyssop, Frankincense, Myrrh, Spikenard, Galbanum, Cinnamon, Calamus, and Olive as a base.

The resultant product is a blend that may create a protective barrier against harmful germs and viruses. *The Essential Oils Desk Reference* (EODR) has this to say about Exodus II™:

> "Some researchers believe that these aromatics were used by Moses to protect the Israelites from a plague. Modern science shows that these oils contain either immune-stimulating or antiviral compounds or both, which may explain why these oils were used in ancient times. Today viruses and bacteria are beginning to mutate and become resistant to conventional drugs. Because of the complex chemistry of essential oils, viruses and bacteria have a more difficult time acquiring resistance." (EODR, 2nd edition, p. 96)

Oils vs. Antibiotics

The statement quoted above from the EODR mentions mutating microbes that resist conventional drugs. This leads us to discuss a major difference in the actions of oils and those of commercial antibiotics in fighting germs.

The reason resistant strains of bacteria develop is because of antibiotic drugs. They cause them. What happens is that when an antibiotic is used and billions of bacteria are killed, one or two may survive. Eventually, these one or two can multiply until there are billions of them that are resistant to or unaffected by the antibiotic that stimulated their creation.

In response, pharmaceutical companies continually strive to develop new, more powerful antibiotics that can destroy the resistant strains. But until such antibiotics are developed, the resistant bacteria can attack and make us sick and we are defenseless. Some such strains are so virulent that they can be fatal. Virtually all of these strains live in hospitals where massive amounts of antibiotics of every variety are administered every day. This fact makes hospitals the most infectious places in the community, posing hazards even to visitors.

The reason that bacteria can become resistant to specific antibiotics is because an antibiotic drug consists of a specific chemical makeup and is identical in every batch that is manufactured. This consistency of product is called "pharmacological purity" and is something in which drug companies take pride. They want a physician using their product to know that when he or she prescribes a drug, it is going to be exactly the same year in and year out, without fail.

Another reason for consistency in manufacturing is research. In order to conduct research under the usual rules of science, the variables must be controlled as much as possible. By having identical batches of a given medicine every time it is produced, you have removed one variable. You know that the patients you test today for a given drug are receiving the very same drug you used in testing last month or ten years ago. Medical scientists don't like to test things like oils because they introduce an uncontrollable variable into the equation.

Unfortunately, the "purity" of synthetically or commercially produced drugs is also their Achilles heel. It is their weakness. Because of the predictability and consistency of every batch of a specific antibiotic, the bacteria eventually learn to recognize it and adapt in ways that protect them and make them resistant.

The very characteristic that doctors, research scientists, and the pharmaceutical companies value the most is the very characteristic that makes all antibiotics eventually useless. It is only a matter of time before the secrets of every antibiotic are unraveled by the intelligence of the bacteria they were designed to attack. Then the bacteria begin winning out, another battle is lost, and the antibiotic is no longer effective.

Why Don't Drug Companies Sell Oils?

The main reason drug companies don't produce or sell essential oils is because they can't be patented to create a profitable monopoly. Anyone with the knowledge and wherewithal to invest can grow aromatic plants and distill oils from them.

Some companies try to produce synthetic versions of essential oils, manufacturing the main components of, say, lavender, and then combine the ingredients to make a fake lavender. The problem is that while such oils may have a fragrance satisfactory for perfumes, aftershave lotions, deodorants and shampoos, they have no healing properties. Only an oil made by God has that.

Therefore, another reason pharmaceuticals don't deal with therapeutic oils is because the only way they can be produced is to let nature make them. When nature makes things, she never does it quite the same way twice.

Essential oils are like fine wines. Even when harvested from the same fields, each year's crop is slightly different because no two years ever have quite the same sunlight, temperature, wind, and rain conditions. And, of course, oils grown in different fields, in different countries, climates, or continents can vary greatly even though they may all be from the same species of plant.

With a product whose chemistry is never quite the same, pharmaceutical companies cannot produce the consistent "purity" upon which they rest their reputations. Neither can a physician using the product know if this month's supply of frankincense or basil oil is like last month's. In fact, he or she can count on it not being the same. Furthermore, controlled studies, which are possible with manufactured drugs, are impossible with natural oils because you never have quite the same material with which to test patients.

A Drug's Weakness is an Oil's Strength

The endless and unpredictable variation in the composition of a particular species of oil that is considered so undesirable and disadvantageous to druggists and doctors is, in fact, one of the most desirable and advantageous qualities of an essential oil. Because of their variability and unpredictability, bacteria can never anticipate ways to resist an essential oil. Therefore, resistance to essential oils can never develop. Oils that were effective against bacteria in Egypt and Israel thousands of years ago are just as effective today as they ever were. Their effectiveness will never diminish even thousands of years hence.

As for antibiotics, the days are numbered for every one of them. Doctors have always known this. Some day, when bacteria become resistant to the final and most potent of antibiotics man can produce, then the use of antibiotics in medicine will be over. It will be history—a temporary measure of the medical system during the twentieth and twenty-first centuries. These are the decades when using antibiotics will come to a permanent end. So you need to be looking for alternatives. And the best one is essential oils.

While a variety of essential oils are effective against fighting bacteria and do so in a way that microbes will never be able to develop resistance, essential oils also have another advantage. Many are virucides.

Antibiotics have no effect on viruses. When they are effective, it is only against bacteria. Hence, antibiotics can never be a cure for the flu or the common cold. Many people have already found that oils help support their immune systems against the common viral infections that visit us annually in their seasons. These people need no double-blind studies to verify their experience. Their experience is sufficient proof.

Antibiotics are Robots . . Essential Oils are Alive

Another important difference between the actions of oils and antibiotics is their intelligence. A true therapeutic grade essential oil is smart. It can tell the bad guys from the good ones. Our bodies function normally and in health with the help of millions of friendly bacteria that live in our intestines and elsewhere in our bodies.

Antibiotics kill off everything indiscriminantly, unable to tell one bacteria from another. They are microscopic killing machines, programmed to seek out bacteria without discrimination. In other words, they are brainless robots. They are made by fallible men.

Aromatic oils know the difference between the bacteria we need and the hostile invaders. They kill off only the invaders, leaving the friendly flora intact. They are made by our infallible God and imbued with his benevolent intelligence.

When we use antibiotics to overcome a bacterial infection, we are left in a weakened state. Our immune systems have been compromised. Until we can re-establish a new culture of friendly bacteria in our bodies, we are more susceptible to the next illness that comes along.

When we use oils to fight bad bacteria, our systems come out stronger. Our immune systems have been strengthened. Our beneficial bacteria have been left untouched. We are better able to deal with the next barrage of disease-causing germs that may appear.

Antibiotics in an Emergency

Antibiotics can sometimes work faster than oils in making the symptoms of a present disease disappear, but in the long run, they will also do you harm. Always. There are no effective drugs without negative side effects.

But when oils, herbs, and other medicines created by God are used, there are usually no negative side effects. In fact, sometimes when you address one medical problem (such as cancer) using natural means, the side effects may be that another condition (like diabetes) disappears as well. Or when one uses various oils to deal with emotional conditions (such as depression), another ailment (like arthritis) may be relieved as an unexpected side effect. Such are the blessings of using medicine created by God instead of the false medicines manufactured by man.

We are not saying that there is no place for antibiotics. When a genuine medical emergency exists and the threat of death is near, a shot of antibiotics may save your life when the use of oils might act too slowly. But their benefits are only temporary. True healing, which would be in the form of a strengthened immune system, must come from another source.

So use your discretion at all times. And please consult with a licensed health care provider when you make your decisions. There is a time and place for antibiotics. You will have to be the judge.

Using Exodus II

Exodus II can be applied by anointment (i.e. rubbed on the skin) through which the oils are absorbed into the body transdermally. It can be breathed through the nose and into the lungs where it enters the brain and blood stream directly. It can also be taken orally in small quantities, 1-2 drops at a time, mixed with a few drops of vegetable oil. By ingestion the healing molecules enter our systems via the absorbent tissues of the mouth and the gastrointestinal tract. Biblical people used oils all three ways.

Exodus II, and all other essential oils, should be used with caution and common sense. Some people have sensitive skin and everyone has sensitive skin in certain areas. So add some vegetable or massage oil when you rub it on. If it starts to heat or turn red, put on more vegetable oil and it will stop. This will not dilute the effective action of the oil. It simply slows down the rate of absorption and relieves the heat.

It must also be kept in mind that everyone's body and emotional makeup are different. Hence, the effects of any particular oil or blend of oils are not totally predictable. The response depends on the individual. While untoward reactions are rare, some people may respond with what seems to be an allergenic reaction. If a person is prone to allergies or has other medical conditions that could predispose them to a reaction, they should consult a health care professional, as well as a knowledgeable aromatherapist, before trying any essential oil.

See the *Essential Oils Desk Reference* or Higley's *Reference Guide for Essential Oils* for more detailed information on using Exodus II and other oils.

Regardless of how they are used, Biblical oils have powerful properties. No doubt they helped keep the Aaronic priesthood of the Israelites free from many diseases. While the holy blends were not available to the people at large, the component oils were. Cinnamon, hyssop, and cassia, for example, are powerful antiseptics, while myrrh can also be used for a variety of therapeutic purposes. Any one of the oils of Exodus can be used alone with healing benefits.

Immune to the Black Plague

Another formula available commercially, which is just as effective and less expensive than Exodus II™ is a blend called Thieves™. These two blends may be considered as having similar actions and can sometimes be used for the same purposes.Thieves contains cinnamon, which is one of the most active ingredients in Exodus II as well as in the holy anointing oil of Exodus 30.

The name "Thieves" comes from its interesting history. During the Dark Ages of Europe there were several great plagues that killed millions. These fatal epidemics were so contagious that when people died, no one was willing to remove the bodies for fear of contracting the illness themselves. People would fall dead in the street and be left untouched and unburied.

However, there were some thieves who stripped these bodies of their jewelry and broke into the homes of the deceased to rob them and they didn't get sick. When a king arrested several of them, he demanded their secret upon pain of death.

The king discovered that these robbers were actually perfumers and spice traders who knew about the protective properties of essential oils. They used oils such as clove, cinnamon, lemon, eucalyptus, and rosemary which they rubbed on their bodies and put on masks for breathing. Thus, came the name "Thieves" for this highly effective blend.

The King who arrested the thieves and made this discovery was King James, the one who commissioned the English translation of the *Bible* in 1611.

Scientific Testing

Thieves™ has been tested at Weber State University for its potent antimicrobial properties. Thieves was found to have a 99.96% kill rate against airborne bacteria. Cinnamon bark oil, which is in Exodus II, has been tested alongside the antibiotics, penicillin and ampicillin, in their effectiveness against *Escherichia coli* and *Staphylococcus aureus*. The effectiveness of cinnamon was found to be comparable to the antibiotics for both types of bacteria. This data is published in the second edition of the *Essential Oils Desk Reference* (EODR) on page 411.

Thieves™ and Exodus II™ can be used in the same ways for the similar results. During the cold and flu seasons, they can both be applied to the soles of one's feet (or one's children's feet) without diluting them. Doing this before going to work or before sending your little ones to school may support the immune system and reduce the chances of catching whatever bugs may be floating around. One can also diffuse either of these oils in the home upon return from work or after school to create an unwelcome environment for any bugs that may have entered from being in contact with the outside world.

The advantage of Thieves is its price, which is not quite so precious as the cost of Exodus II. The advantage of Exodus II is that it is milder, less prone to burn sensitive skin, and has spiritual and emotional benefits. It is also scripturally based on oils and formulas given by God, himself, and used by his chosen people.

Oils for Courage and Spiritual Awakening

Another blend of oils of scriptural origin commercially available is called "3 Wise Men™." It contains the following oils:

Sandalwood (Aloes), Myrrh, Juniper, Frankincense, Spruce, and Almond oil as a base.

All of these oils were used in Biblical times, including oils of spruce and almond. *The Essential Oils Desk Reference* (EODR) has this to say about 3 Wise Men™:

> This blend was formulated to open the subconscious mind through pineal stimulation to help release deep-seated trauma. These oils bring a sense of grounding and uplifting through emotional releasing and elevated spiritual consciousness. (EODR, 2nd edition, p. 124)

The reference to "pineal" stimulation has to do with the fact that when aromatic molecules are inhaled, they not only pass down into our lungs and reach the blood stream, they also travel by way of the olfactory nerves directly into the center of the brain where forgotten emotional trauma is stored. More is discussed on this aspect of how oils work to heal us in the chapter entitled "Oils of Joy." You may also want to refer back to the section entitled "Oils and Emotions" in Chapter Two, "How and Why Oils Can Heal."

Spruce is an ingredient in the 3 Wise Men™ blend mentioned above. While reference to spruce oil is not found anywhere in scripture, it was in use in Biblical times. There is a blend of oils containing spruce called "Valor™." It has the emotional impact of stimulating courage. It contains the following:

> Rosewood, Blue Tansy, Frankincense, and Spruce in a carrier base oil of Almond.

All of these oils were in use during Biblical times, especially by the Romans, prior to and during the time of Christ. The EODR has this to say about Valor™:

> Valor helps balance electrical energies within the body, giving courage, confidence, and self-esteem. It has been found to help the body self-correct its balance and alignment giving relief of pain. The oils in this blend empower the physical and spiritual bodies to overcome fear and opposition when facing adversity. It helps build courage, confidence, and self-esteem. Valor has been touted as a "chiropractor in a bottle." It has improved scoliosis for

some in as little as 30 minutes, while other individuals require several applications. Valor has also been shown to change anaerobic-mutated cells back to their aerobic natural state. (EODR, 2nd edition, p. 126)

The formulation of Valor™ came from studying the oils used by Roman soldiers before going into battle. More than 2,000 years ago the Romans discovered that these oils could be applied to their feet and shoulders and it would give them courage. With such fearlessness, they conquered the Western World.

One of the properties of this blend is that it can stimulate the spine to self-correct, sometimes even by just smelling it briefly. It is this property that gave it the nickname of "chiropractor in a bottle."

There is a technique of anointment with oils called "raindrop" where Valor is applied at the beginning and at the end. People normally grow from 1/8 to 1/2 inch during the procedure, which takes about an hour. Occasionally, people grow an inch or more. According to the *Essential Oils Desk Reference*, raindrop technique "has resolved numerous cases of scoliosis and kyphosis and eliminated the need for back surgery for thousands of people." (EODR, p. 191)

However it works, this oil can cause one to stand more erect, increasing the length of one's backbone. If you think about it, what is courage anyhow? Is it not also referred to as "having backbone?"

As an instructor and facilitator of raindrop technique myself, I have anointed people with raindrop oils many times and have seen Valor™ do its magic hundreds of times. So I speak from personal experience on this point. (See page 325 on The Raindrop Study.)

Anointing to Heal as Taught by Christ

In Mark's Gospel, we read of Jesus sending out his twelve disciples in pairs to minister to the public. As they prepared to depart, Jesus gave them the following instructions:

"In what place soever ye enter into an house and there abide till ye depart from that place. And whosoever shall not receive you, nor hear you, when ye depart thence, shake off the dust under your feet for a testimony against them. Verily I say unto you, It shall be more tolerable for Sodom and Gomorrha in the day of judgment than for that city." (Mark 6:10-11)

The same instructions are also given in Luke 10:1-12. These passages from Mark and Luke are packed with Divine direction for us. First of all, Jesus did not heal just anyone. He healed only those who were receptive to him and in almost every instance when the healing had been accomplished he said, "Thy faith had made thee whole." He never once said, "I have healed thee." The *New Testament* relates only a sample of the thousands of healings Jesus must have facilitated in his brief ministry, but in no instance in the Biblical record did Jesus just approach an ailing stranger and say, "Here let me heal you." In every case the blind, the lame, and the afflicted (or their friends and relatives) came to Jesus in faith, believing that they or their loved one would be healed through him.

That point is made clearly in these passages where Jesus basically says, "Go where you are accepted, welcomed, and greeted in friendship because you can help these people. They are receptive. But where you are greeted with resistance, doubt, or disbelief, don't waste your time. Move on. And when you go, don't look back or grieve over them. They have chosen to miss a wonderful opportunity to be made whole in body, mind and spirit through your loving ministry, and they have turned it down in prejudice and ignorance. They will suffer greatly for their mistake and you can't help them. So go on."

This passage carries an important practical lesson for those of us who understand the blessings God has provided through the gift of essential oils and want to share it. The lesson is this:

Shake the Dust Off Your Feet and Leave

When you find people who need the healing therapies that essential oils can bring, and they resist you or ridicule you and reject your offerings made in good faith, move on. If they are not receptive to these healing concepts at this time, you can't help them.

Don't try to convince them. You can't. Their inability to see and understand what a great gift you offer is not an intellectual thing that can be corrected with more facts. It is a spiritual and emotional thing. They will just have to suffer.

You can love them and pray for them, but until they come to you voluntarily on their own, with an open heart, you can't help them. It is a waste of your time and an imposition on theirs, as well. Spend your time seeking those who are receptive and ready. Those people you can help.

That is the message Jesus has for us in these two passages. And that is the example he set in his own ministry. The quotation from Mark comes right after Jesus visited Nazareth where he had grown up as a boy, and found himself rejected as an adult. When stories of his miracles were heard by the townsfolk from abroad, all they could think was, "Is not this the son of the carpenter? Is not this the son of Mary and the brother of James, Joses, Juda, and Simon? And are not his sisters here, also?" They were offended by what seemed to them to be exaggerated stories of his powers and arrogance on the part of Jesus not to deny them. In his home town, he was just another guy, not a Messiah with miraculous powers.

"A prophet is not without honor," remarked Jesus, "except in his own country, among his own kin, and in his own house." (Mark 6:4)

Jesus marveled at their unbelief and sadly left town, unable to do any great works in that place which had been his home. But there is more.

Causes of Sickness

The next two verses of this passage in Mark contain a lot of information concentrated in a few words:

"And they went out, and preached that men should repent. And they cast out many devils, and anointed with oil many that were sick, and healed them." (Mark 6:12-13)

The first phrase of this text is crucial to healing, "that men should repent." This verse implies that when one is sick due to a long engagement in unhealthy activities (such as alcohol abuse or the use of tobacco), in order to be healed there must come a change (repentance) in the lifestyle that produced that illness (like giving up the alcohol or tobacco). While sickness can certainly come as a result of our own actions—i.e., lung cancer from smoking, diabetes from poor food choices, and nervous conditions from too much worry and too little faith in the Lord—not all sickness is from personal transgressions of health laws. Let's discuss those kinds of sicknesses first.

Some illnesses are from environmental factors outside of our control, such as contracting cancer from working in a factory for years and breathing asbestos we did not even know was there. Some injuries or disabilities are the result of accidents for which we were not responsible, like being hit head-on by a drunk driver.

Sometimes illness comes as a genetic hand-me-down we could not and would not have chosen. Some consider such illnesses to be generational curses. (Exodus 20:5, Deuteronomy 5:9)

Sometimes illness can even come by God's permission as a test of our faith. Job was an example of this kind of sickness where Satan was allowed to afflict him with boils to test his trust in God. (Job 2:1-3)

Sometimes a person is afflicted with a disability as part of a greater Divine plan. An example of this is the man born without sight mentioned in John 9:1-3. When Jesus' disciples asked if the man's blindness was because of his sins or because of those of his parents, Jesus replied, "Neither hath this man sinned, nor his parents: but that the works of God should be made manifest in him." Jesus thereupon healed the man of his blindness. This man was then to play a key role in the developing issues between

Jesus and the Pharisees that ultimately led to the cross. (John 9:8-38)

Our response to a disease inflicted by God for spiritual purposes is one thing. But most of our problems cannot be attributed to God. In many cases our sicknesses are caused by our own thoughts, emotions, and actions by what we eat, breathe, drink, and do on a daily basis. Somehow, in some way, we have failed to obey some of God's natural or spiritual laws for maintaining wellness.

Sickness may come as a wake-up call for us to stop, introspect, figure out what we may have done to get ourselves into this situation, and then repent—that is, make whatever changes are necessary in our lifestyles to remedy the problem and prevent it from happening again. Every illness is an opportunity to correct past mistakes, acquire new wisdom, make spiritual progress, increase in righteousness, and grow closer to God.

This is a hard thing for many people to accept—the idea that they may be, to one extent or another, personally responsible for many of the illnesses they suffer. They would rather believe that they suffer heart disease, diabetes, fibromyalgia, arthritis, cancer, etc., because they are random victims of fate. The *Bible* suggests otherwise. "The curse causeless does not come." (Proverbs 26:2)

Some illness may well be randomly assigned. We can't do much about that. But the illnesses we have played a part in creating, that we can do something about by understanding our part, admitting responsibility, and changing our ways, (in other words, by repenting).

A More Excellent Way

There is a wonderful book entitled, *A More Excellent Way*, by Pastor Henry Wright. The title comes from the last words of the twelfth chapter of I Corinthians which immediately precede St. Paul's well known "Love Chapter." Rev. Wright has one of the most successful healing ministries in the Christian world. He is the senior pastor of the Pleasant Valley Church in Thomaston, Georgia, but his healing ministry is worldwide. Rev. Wright says that many sicknesses come from negative emotions like unforgiveness, revenge, bitterness, envy, pride, jealousy, resentment, anger, or hatred. Feelings of a poor self image can be destructive to our physical and mental health.

When a healing is sought at the Pleasant Valley Church, Rev. Wright, or one of his staff members, first probes into your spiritual life to find the emotions, feelings and spiritual issues that you have not resolved and continue to harbor. They do that before they ever pray for the remission of your illness. This is because they know from experience that until you have cleared (repented of) any bitterness that may underlie your sickness, prayer is not likely to be effective. (Visit <www.PleasantValleyChurch.net> for more information.)

Why Prayer Doesn't Always Work

When we suffer with a disease, even a fatal one, there is often a part of us that wants to be healed but another part that does not. Sickness can serve to bring us some of the things we want in life, like sympathy or a sense of self-worth or freedom from certain responsibilities because we are sick. Sickness is often an unconscious choice at an emotional level. We have actually invited the disease into our lives without knowing it. When the opportunity comes to be healed, we may accept it consciously and intellectually, but reject it subconsciously and emotionally.

Extreme examples of this are hypocondriacs who spend small fortunes on doctors, drugs, and procedures, but never get any better. They relish the attention and sympathy they receive. They like being able to talk about their trials, pains, and "rare" ailments to everyone they meet. They enjoy the fact that "being chronically sick" relieves them of many responsibilities. The incredible amount of money being spent on them (thanks to insurance and government programs) gives them a sense of value and enhances their self-image. But it is a false self-image, not the divine image of God we were intended to manifest. For such people, prayer is useless. Even Jesus didn't try to heal such persons.

Without getting to the root cause of your sickness to remove the emotional and spiritual barriers you have placed between you and God's grace, prayers will be ineffective. Without genuine repentance, your prayers are like asking for God's help with your words and thoughts while blocking his help with your feelings and emotions. Your appeal for divine intervention is mixed and contradictory— asking God to remove a problem verbally while clinging to the problem emotionally. This is why God often does not seem to answer prayer.

God Always Answers Prayer

The truth is, God always responds exactly to the messages we send to him. It is just that the messages we send are usually self-nullifying contradictions. We want something without the willingness to prepare ourselves to receive it. We want God to plant the seed, but we aren't willing to prepare the soil or nurture the plant.

When we are sick we pray, "God please heal me. . . but not yet. I still want to hang on to these hidden emotions and attitudes that are the cause of my sickness." God's answer is, "Okay. Go ahead. Hang on to them. When you are ready to let go, repent, clean up your bitter thoughts, change your negative habits, accept full responsibility for what you are doing to yourself, forgive those who have hurt you, stop blaming others for your problems—then call me again. Until then, I can't heal you." That is God's answer, which perfectly fits the self-contradicting prayer we have sent to him. James 4:3 says it nicely: "Ye ask, and receive not, because ye ask amiss."

As his children, God has given us free will. God respects you too much to heal you against your will. When both your conscious and unconscious will are in alignment with God and you ask him for healing with all of your heart, body, mind, spirit and soul, on all levels, both conscious and unconscious, then you will be healed. This is what constitutes faith. This is the kind of faith Jesus described in Matthew 17:20 and Mark 11:23,

We Can Fool Ourselves, but Not God

You see, when we send a prayer to God, he gets the whole message, not just the verbal or outward prayer, but the emotions, too, including those hidden even to ourselves. We can hide our true selves from ourselves, but we can't hide it from God. To pray effectively, we must work to become aware of our deepest feelings and, through forgiveness and understanding, accept them and let them go. Essential oils are a great help in this regard. They can awaken forgotten emotions and bring them to our conscious minds so we can know the truth about ourselves, give it to God, deal with it, and be free.

John 8:43 says it well: "Ye shall know the truth, and the truth shall make you free." Among other interpretations, this scripture perfectly describes the liberating transformation from sickness to health we can experience by bringing the truth of our hidden emotions into conscious awareness so we can "know" and deal with them. Sometimes this can be painful, but in order to be free we have to accept the pain and pass through it. When we are willing to do that, we can be healed, and prayer will work. When we are both emotionally and intellectually ready, healing by prayer can be instantaneous and permanent.

If you want to learn more about the ministry of the Pleasant Valley Church, call (800) 453-5775 and order Pastor Wright's book. It's over 300 pages long and packed full of healing wisdom from the scriptures.

Repentance is an Ongoing Attitude

The point of this discussion is to explain why in Mark 6:12 we read that when Jesus sent his disciples out to heal, the healing was to be preceded by repentance. We want you to understand that this repentance was something much bigger than just saying "I'm sorry." It is much more than saving one's soul for a better life after death.

Jesus' ministry was to also show people how they could be whole and healthy while still in this mortal body before they die.

Repentance is the state of mind necessary to be open to God's healing power regardless of whether the healing be via the vehicle of prayer or via the vehicle of His medicines or both. Repentance is an attitude of willingness to accept full responsibility for one's condition, willingness to make the effort to correct the ignorance that led to that condition, and resolve to change one's lifestyle and not commit the same error again. Repentance is not something we do once. It is a state of openness and appreciation to God we must maintain on a daily basis. Repentance is a state of humility that accepts God as the sole source of healing and is the necessary foundation by which we can receive his grace. (II Chronicles 7:14)

All of the people that Jesus healed in the *Bible* were, at some level, humble, repentant and receptive—ready to receive his healing blessings. The unreceptive and the unrepentant, Jesus could not help and did not try. That is why he didn't seek to heal pharisees. He would have, but they were not open to receive Him. They remained unrepentant to the end.

How permanent were Jesus's healings? We don't know. Whether some of those whom Christ healed backslid, unable to maintain their repentant attitude indefinitely, we can't say. The *Bible* doesn't provide us with any followup histories. How long a healing lasts probably depends on the person. If they fall back into the habits that caused their illness, they may be sick again. Repentance is necessary to receive from God. Continued repentance is necessary to maintain and keep that which God has given.

Casting Out Devils

The first part of Mark 6:12-13 was about repentance and its relationship to disease and healing. The second part has to do with demons and unclean spirits. Many modern Christians don't believe in demonic possession. But Jesus and his disciples did and so do I. A large percent of Jesus' healings involved the casting out of devils. Look up the following scriptures and you will see: Matthew 4:24; 8:16, 28. 33; 9:32; 12:22; 15:22; Mark 1:32; 5:15, 16, 18; 16:17; Luke 4:33, 41; 8:36. This is just a sample of the references to devils, demons and evil spirits. There are more.

St. Paul describes the situation perfectly in his letter to the Ephesians:

"For we wrestle not against flesh and blood, but against principalities, against powers, against the rulers of the darkness of this world, against spiritual wickedness in high places." (Ephesians 6:12)

If you have no conscious experience in encountering demonic possessions, then you may find no basis to believe in them. It is one of Satan's cleverest tricks to influence us not to believe in him nor his army of demonic assistants.

The point is that when engaged in a healing mission, one must be ready to deal with all aspects of disease. Some sicknesses are of demonic origin. Rev. Wright has discovered this by experience and deals with it in his book.

Demonic spirits don't like essential oils. They are repelled by them. Their high vibrations, put there by God, are too much and make them want to leave. Those experienced in the administration of therapeutic oils, especially when used to help resolve and release buried emotions, can find themselves encountering demons repulsed by the high energies of the aromatic molecules. This is not likely to happen, but if it does, know that by the power of God and the Holy Spirit you will be guided as to what to do. Intense prayer and calling on the name of Jesus Christ will always prevail in such situations.

As a last comment on casting out evil spirits, consider this passage from Matthew:

"When an unclean spirit has gone out of a person, it wanders through waterless regions looking for a resting place, but it finds none. Then it says, 'I will return to my house from which I came.' When it comes, it finds it empty, swept, and put in order. Then it goes and brings along seven other spirits more evil than itself, and they enter and live there; and the last state of that person is worse than the first." (Matthew 12:43-45)

In other words, when you have been cleared of a possession, you must fill the void with righteousness. To make the healing permanent, you must repent and adapt your lifestyle toward greater spirituality.

Demons of Our Own Making

There are also "demons" that are not the independent and conscious entities described in the *New Testament* to whom Jesus spoke as if they were personalities. Some of these Biblical devils or demons would be properly diagnosed, according to modern psychiatry, as neuroses or psychoses. These are "demons" or "unclean spirits" of our own making—psychological disorders, hang-ups, and psychiatric diseases, that hide our true selves and prevent the flow of God's love into our lives.

Both kinds of demons, those conscious entities from the unseen realms of darkness spoken of by Paul in Ephesians and those of our own making, need to be dealt with and "cast out" in order to affect a healing. Scientifically trained psychologists, psychotherapists, and psychiatrists tend to disbelieve in conscious demonic entities and try to explain everything in terms of personal psychology or biochemistry. The limited secular view of such professionals has its validity, but their paradigm is incomplete. Jesus dealt with devils as real personalities, talking with them and ordering them out.

Jesus' instructions to his disciples for healing, as found in the Gospels, were only a few words (summarized in Mark 6:7-13), but they covered every aspect of sickness and healing, including the demonic and the release of demon-like mental disorders.

Anointing with Oil

In Mark 6:13 Jesus instructs his disciples to anoint the sick with oils and heal them. Mark does not elaborate on the content of the oils used by the disciples. Mark didn't explain this passage because he knew that his readers of that day would have known that it was customary for "anointing oils" to contain aromatic ingredients. When an anointing oil was referred to simply as "oil," it was understood by the people of that time that the vegetable oil was only a carrier for the vital essences of the aromatics it contained. Using a vegetable base as a carrier allowed the disciples to use their stock of essential oils more cost effectively and enable them to share them with more people.

Gradual Healing vs. Instant Healing

One can get the impression from reading the *New Testament* that all of the healings of Jesus and his disciples were "instantaneous." But this was not so. There are three Greek words translated as "healing" in the *New Testament*, all with different meanings.

The healing Greek word "iaomai" does mean "miraculous" or "instantaneous" and is found 30 times in the *New Testament*. (cf. Matthew 8:13; Mark 5:29; Luke 8:47; John 12:40) However, the Greek word "therapeuo," from which we get our word "therapy," is found 40 times in the *New Testament*. (cf. Matthew 4:23-24; Mark 1:34; Luke 5:15; Acts 5:16, 8:7). Therapeuo means, literally, "to serve, to attend to, or to wait upon menially" or in other words, "to heal gradually over time with care."

Sometimes prayer, anointing, and healing needs to occur in stages over a period of time accompanied by a physical attendant to "care for the sick." Such healings are no less miraculous. They just aren't instantaneous. In Acts 28:8 Paul performs an instantaneous healing (iaomai) while in the very next verse (28:9) he performs other healings (therapeuo) that were not instantaneous requiring the loving care of a friend or relative for a time.

The third Greek word for healing in the *Scriptures* is "sozo," which is found only three times. (Mark 5:23; Luke 8:36; Acts 14:9) Sozo implies not only a physical healing, but an emotional and spiritual one as well. Literally, sozo means "to become sound or whole" in body, mind and spirit.

In Mark 6:13 where Jesus instructs his disciples to "anoint the sick with oil and heal them," the healing word is "therapeuo."

An Experience with Both Kinds of Healing

In the introduction of this book (pp. xxiii–xxiv) I describe a personal experience of instantaneous healing from 43 years of back pain with one session of prayerfully laying on of hands and anointing with oils. It was a miracle. It was iaomai. I have also experienced therapeuo.

I severely injured my right knee back in 1964. I was 27 at the time. It hurt for ten years. I thought the pain would never stop, but it did. The knee was fine until the year 2000 when I passed the age of 63. Suddenly it began to develop a severe osteoarthritis. It hurt with every step. I limped from the pain. And it ached all night, disrupting my sleep. I couldn't run or jump without the knee swelling up and the pain getting even worse. The doctor said the only remedy would be a knee replacement. I said "No thanks."

I then prayed for guidance and was led to apply cypress and wintergreen oils. I also added Panaway™ oil, mixing three drops of each oil in my hand and rubbing them over my knee morning and evening, with prayer. I started receiving relief right away, and gradually the knee began to mend. After two months of daily anointing it was completely healed. That was several years ago, and I am still running and jumping with no pain. That was therapeuo. Although it was not instantaneous, it was, to me, no less of a miracle.

This example illustrates how you determine the oils to use in any given situation and how to apply them. You simply ask God, the master aromatherapist and master healer. If you listen, he will inform you. "Ask, and it shall be given you; seek and you shall find." (Matthew 7:7) "You do not have, because you do not ask. You ask and receive not, because you ask wrongly." (James 4:2-3) "Be still and know that I am God." (Psalm 46:10)

Why Not Just Prayer?

Jesus not only taught his disciples that prayer and repentance was part of the healing procedure, he also taught the use of oils. Since the New Testament does not explain much about which oils are to be used, many have interpreted that to mean that it doesn't matter. They believe that the oil is of symbolic or ritualistic value only, and that plain olive, or just any old oil, will do. Some churches have even used mineral oil, which is a petroleum product and potentially harmful. Some Christians reject the idea of healing oils altogether, remarking that "Prayer is enough. You don't need oils."

As discussed on pages xvii-xviii of the introduction, essential oils are special creations of God, infused with his Word. (Genesis 1:11-12, John 1:1) Being the products of God's words and thoughts, they respond to our words and thoughts. Essential oils magnify intent. Stop and read that again. Essential oils magnify intent. When we apply them and mentally or verbally direct them to places in the body that need therapy, the oils respond to your thoughts and understand. They will go where you have directed and administer their healing vibrations. When we pray over oils, their frequencies increase. When their electromagnetic frequencies increase, so does their ability to uplift and heal. When our intent is expressed as prayer, oils amplify that intent and increase the effectiveness of the prayer.

Prayer can work without oils. Oils can work without prayer. When both are used together, each increases the power of the other such that their combined ability to heal is greater than the sum of the two. This is no coincidence. It was programmed into the oils by God from their creation. Prayer and oils were meant to be used together.

If you are having success with prayer alone, it can be increased by the intelligent use of oils. If you are having success with oils, apply them with prayer and you will see even greater success.

Sold Out to Secular Medicine

Many Christians who reject God's oils as medicine on the basis that prayer is better and sufficient are totally sold out to the medical profession as if it were their church. They will religiously pay their insurance premi-

ums before they pay their tithe. While they may forget to
pray regularly every day, they would never forget to take
their daily prescriptions. While they may miss church from
time to time, they would never miss a doctor's appoint-
ment or a visit to the hospital recommended by their doctor. When they are sick, do they follow the advice of James
5:14 and go to the church to be anointed and healed by the
elders? No. They go to the hospital to be infused with pharmaceuticals by medical staff. And when a medical emergency arises, their first impulse is to call an ambulance or
911 instead of praying to God to receive his guidance in
the matter of whether 911 should be called or if, perhaps,
there is a better course to take.

Such people, who consider themselves Christians,
exhibit more faith in secular medicine than in God and
prayer, yet they object to God's medicine (oils), saying that
prayer is sufficient and they don't need oils. Why do such
people place their belief in commercial drugs designed by
corporations whose motive is to maximize profits? Why
don't they place their belief in natural medicines designed
by God whose only motive, as a loving Father, is for our
happiness and well-being.

God's means of healing sometimes requires medicines.
The best medicines are the ones he made. Among the best
of these are the aromatic oils of the plant kingdom. God's
medicines work better when accompanied with prayer, and
prayer works better when accompanied with God's medicines. It isn't one or the other. Both are gifts from the same
source. Both were meant by their provider for us to use,
and to use intelligently—and that means always with his
guidance.

Where's the Money?

One may wonder how Jesus (who was not a wage
earner during the years of his ministry) and his disciples (who gave up their means of income when they
chose to follow) could afford precious ointments. An
answer is suggested in Luke's Gospel:

"And it came to pass afterward, that he went throughout every city and village, preaching and showing the glad tidings of the kingdom of God: and the twelve were with him, And certain women, which had been healed of evil spirits and infirmities, Mary called Magdalene, out of whom went seven devils, And Joanna the wife of Chuza Herod's steward, and Susanna, and many others, which ministered unto him of their substance." (Luke 8:1-3)

Jesus' ministry was underwritten financially by his women followers and the resources (substance) available to them. Is this not like today where, for many churches, it is the women who raise the money and support the missions of the church? Add to this that Jesus had many wealthy friends (Nicodemus, Lazarus, Joseph of Arimathea) not to mention that several of his twelve disciples were also affluent or well-to-do, such as Matthew the tax collector, and the businessmen, John, James, Peter, and Andrew, who owned a fleet of fishing boats. Jesus was able to attract whatever money he needed, and his store of precious oils was probably kept by some of his women followers, acting as superintendents of his treasury.

Jesus and his disciples did have the means to afford a supply of aromatic oils. The Holy Land itself was a major producer of essential oils from its own indigenous vegetation. It was also the major crossroads of the aromatic oil trade of the world. Hence, liquid spices of all kinds were easily available in that time and place. By diluting them in olive oil, the disciples stretched them as far as they could to reach as many as they could. It is incorrect to think that they anointed the sick with a plain cooking oil as a symbol only. There was healing medicine in their oils as well as in their prayers.

Anointing with God's oils, accompanied with prayers for his blessings, is a powerful approach to healing. This is what we believe that Jesus taught and that his disciples did, including the elders of the early church. We want to see this knowledge and this practice return to the sanctuary where it belongs.

Chapter Five
How Many Bible References To Essential Oils?

There are 1,035 references to essential oils, aromatic oil-producing plants, and their applications in the *Bible*, including at least 33 species. This chapter explains in detail how we arrived at these numbers. If statistics and statistical tabulations do not interest you, you may wish to skip to the next chapter, "Oils of Joy." If you are curious about how so many Biblical references to essential oils were discovered and tabulated, then read on.

Essential oils were in daily use by the peoples of the *Bible*—not just by the Israelites and the early Christians. They were used extensively by all the cultures around them, including the Arabians, Assyrians, Phoenicians, Babylonians, Persians, Egyptians, Romans, Greeks, and other cultures around the Mediterranean. Their perfumes, medicines, anointing oils, and incenses all derived their scents, potencies, and healing capabilities from essential oils.

The true extent of the uses and applications of essential oils cannot be determined by the Biblical writings alone because the intent of the writers was not to detail and catalogue herbs and oils, but to present spiritual teachings and their history as it related to God. Hence, the historical and botanical rigor necessary for accurate and complete studies of the oils and aromatic plants of the *Bible* simply isn't there to be tabulated and analyzed in any simple or conclusive way. What is found in the *Bible* is but a sample of the extent to which essential oils were really used in those times and places. From that sample, a great deal can be learned and deduced.

The *Bible* is full of references to essential oils, to their applications, and to the plants from which they were derived. Many references are direct, in that a specific oil is named. Some are indirect, where the name of an oil or plant is not given, but its identity can be deduced. Most references are general, in that no specific oil or oils are named or indicated, but their use is clearly implied.

More than a Simple Word Count

The word oil appears 191 times in the King James Version of the *Bible*. But the answer to the question "How Many *Bible* References to Essential Oils?" is far more than a simple word count. First of all, not all of the mentions of oil fit the definition of an essential or healing oil. (See Chapter Two.) Many of these references are to fatty oils which are not therapeutic. In some cases, we have blends of both types of oils.

One of the most common oils of the *Bible* is virgin or "first" olive oil, which is both an essential oil from the fruit and a fatty oil from the hard seed. Such olive oil has healing properties. So how do we classify aromatic olive oil? Is it essential or fatty? For purposes of tabulating the healing oils of the *Bible*, we choose not to count olive. However, a discussion of olive oil is given in Chapter Eleven. A tabulation of citations for olive oil is given in Appendix D. Only when the olive oil mentioned also contains other aromatics such as cinnamon, cassia, or myrrh, do we count it as a reference to an essential oil.

Getting back to the topic of "How Many *Bible* Oil References?" there are many other complications to consider. Another question that cannot be answered definitively by the *Bible* is, "How many species of plants produced essential oils in Biblical times?" We know from Babylonian, Egyptian, Roman, Greek, and Arabian sources that many oils in use in those days within and around the Hebrew culture are not mentioned in the *Bible*. (See the writings of Tisserand, Rose, and Watt in the Bibliography.) A partial list of unmentioned Biblical oils is given in Appendix C.

There are also oils mentioned in the *Apocrypha* that fill the 400 year historical gap between the last book of the *Old Testament* and the Gospels of the New. Almost all of these oils are also mentioned in the *Bible*, but not all of them. We do not include these in our tabulation for Biblical Oils even though they were used by the people of the *Bible*. Appendix B tabulates the Apocryphal oils.

There is also a problem of identification of species in the *Bible*. The science of accurately distinguishing and naming plant varieties did not exist until the last two centuries. Besides, the *Bible* writers were more focused on religion than on botany. The word "rose" was used by Biblical peoples as a generic term for any brightly colored flowering plant and not just for the thorny, multi-petaled flowering shrub we know as a true rose. (See Chapter Eight on "Roses of the Holy Land.")

Sometimes the *Bible* simply refers to a "gum" or a "resin" without identifying a species. In these cases, unless we can deduce the plant variety from the context, such a reference could be to balm, cistus, galbanum, frankincense, myrrh, or onycha or, perhaps, to several other species.

Corn and Columbus

As for completely wrong identifications given in the *Bible*, consider corn. There are 88 mentions of corn in the *King James Version* of the *Bible*, and every one of them is wrong. Corn is a plant indigenous to North and South America and was unknown in Europe or the Middle East until after Columbus discovered America in 1492. All of the translations since the Authorized KJV of 1881 have substituted the word "grain" wherever the KJV had used "corn."

In the case of anise seed, mentioned in Matthew 23:23 of the KJV, we find that in the *New Revised Standard Version* (NRSV) that verse identifies the seed as dill. Both could be right, since the Greek word used was "anethon," which was a word used for both species at the time. We also know that both dill and anise were sources of essential oil at that time. Anise oil was used medicinally for a variety of purposes, including the cleansing of parasites. Dill oil was given to gladiators to rub on their bodies before then went into the coliseum to fight. The emotional impact of dill oil is to reduce nervousness and make you calm. In this instance where two translations give two different species for the same word, we count them both as oils of the *Bible*, which they were.

Confusion of Words

Other terms than the Greek "anethon" were also used to designate dill in the *Bible*, terms that could be interpreted in various ways. For example, dill is mentioned twice in Isaiah (28:25, 27) in the NRSV whereas in the KJV these passages mention a plant called "fitches" instead. The Hebrew word used by Isaiah was "qetsah," which has three possible translations: dill, black cumin, or an inferior grade of wheat. The term "fitches" also appears in Ezekiel 4:9 (KJV), but here the word chosen is "kussemeth," which is a clear reference to a low grade wheat translated as "spelt" in the NRSV. Since cumin is a fairly straightforward translation from both Hebrew (kammon) and Greek (kuminon), we chose dill as the oil-producing herb mentioned in Isaiah. Hence, we have tabulated three Biblical references to dill: Two in the *Old Testament* and One in the *New*.

References to Plants vs. Oils of Plants

Another problem in tabulating the Biblical references to essential oils is how to tabulate mentions of an actual oil versus mentions of the aromatic plants from which the oils were produced. In references to plants, such as bushes of myrtle or branches of hyssop, it is the aroma (or the essential oil) of the plant that created its appeal and utility to the peoples of the *Bible.*

In cases such as cedar trees, from which cedar oil was distilled, even when used as lumber to build temples, palaces, and synagogues or to manufacture furniture, caskets, or musical instruments—the scent of cedar was always present. Even then the appeal of the building material was its aromatic essential oil.

In some cases we know that plants mentioned only as a plant were also sources of essential oil in that time. (Examples: fir, rose, juniper, shittah, and terebinth.) In these cases, even when mentioned only as an aromatic herb, bush, tree, or flower, we count it as a reference to essential oils, which it truly is.

The foregoing discussion is meant to give you a sample of the kinds of challenges faced in trying to answer the questions of "How Many References to Essential Oils in the *Bible*?" and "How Many Species?" These are simple questions, but they require complex and lengthy answers that can never be exact nor definitive. Nevertheless, useful tabulations can be made, which you will find in this book. They serve as good estimates as to the extent to which essential oils were a part of the daily lives of the peoples of the *Bible*.

Appendix A lists all of the specific, indirect, and general references to essential oils we have so far been able to identify and the numbers are surprising— regardless of the definitions you choose to accept for these tabulations. By the most liberal of interpretations, there are 1035 references to essential oils and the plants from which essential oils were obtained. By even the most restrictive of definitions, there are at least 500 references. So how many references to essential oils are there in the *Bible*? You decide.

What we shall do next is go through the process by which we got our numbers. You may want to refer repeatedly to Appendix A in this discussion.

Citations for Frankincense and Myrrh

Let's start with frankincense and myrrh. These are the two most frequently mentioned healing oils of the *Bible*. The specific word frankincense occurs 16 times in the English *Bible*, but the word "lebonah," which is Hebrew for frankincense, occurs in 6 other places where it was translated as "incense." Hence, there are actually 22 direct references to frankincense by name.

The word myrrh occurs 17 times in the *Bible* plus one reference to stacte in Exodus 30:34, which is another name for myrrh. That gives us 18 direct references to myrrh by name. Adding these together we get 22 + 18 = 40 unequivocal references to these two essential oils in the *Bible*. These are numbers you will find in Tables One-A and Two-A of Appendix A.

But this is only the barest beginning of the count. When we go to Table Three-A we find that indirectly there are 54 references to each Frankincense and to Myrrh as required ingredients for holy incense. This brings our total to 40 + 54 (for Frankincense) + 54 (for myrrh) = 148.

But then we look to the next item in Table Three-A, which is embalming, and find that this adds 4 more each to these two oils. So now we have 148 + 4 (for frankincense) + 4 (for myrrh) = 156.

But we aren't done yet. Looking on the next page of Table Three-A we find that myrrh is always included in the holy anointing oil, and it is mentioned 65 times in the *Bible*. Adding this in we get 156 + 65 = 221.

But wait. In that same table we see that myrrh is translated as "ointment" or "spikenard" 14 times in the *New Testament* when it should have been "myrrh and spikenard" mixed together. (See Chapter Ten.) Adding this in we get: 14 + 221 = 235.

Then add in one more indirect reference for both oils from Exodus 25:6 and you get a grand total of 237 references to frankincense or myrrh in the *Bible*, and this is just two oils. The scores are: 156 for Myrrh and 81 for Frankincense.

Hyssop, Spikenard, and Wormwood

The next most mentioned oil and aromatic herb of the *Bible* is hyssop, mentioned 12 times. (There may be more than one species referred to as hyssop in the *Bible*.) In any case, for the three oils most mentioned by name (myrrh, frankincense, and hyssop)—we have respectively 156 + 81 + 12 = 249.

Spikenard is mentioned five times by name and twice by indirect reference as being in an "alabaster box." Thus, we find 7 references to nard in Table Two-A. In Table Three-A we find 10 additional mentions of spikenard blended with myrrh and referred to as an ointment. Thus, there are 17 references to Spikenard either directly or indirectly. 249 + 17 = 266

Wormwood was another oil used in Biblical times. It is not used in aromatherapy much today. Wormwood has a bitter taste and contains absinthe (thujone), a substance that can cause brain damage and hallucinations if taken internally over an extended time. The people of the *Bible* probably took wormwood oil internally in occasional small amounts as medicine. They were well aware of its bitterness, as well as its toxicity. (Proverbs 5:4; Revelations 8:11) They mostly used the oil in topical ointments and may have eaten some of the leaves as one of the bitter herbs required during the Passover meal. (Exodus 12:8; Numbers 9:11) Wormwood is mentioned 9 times bringing our total now to 266 + 9 = 275.

Balm, Cedarwood, Myrtle, and Aloes

Balm and cedarwood oils are mentioned six times each as is the myrtle tree—from which a healing oil was produced and known for its respiratory and thyroid balancing benefits. This adds another 18 references found in the *Bible*: 18 + 275 = 303 so far.

There is another four indirect references to cedarwood with respect to the Egyptian embalming oils of Genesis listed in Table Three-A. 303 + 4 = 307

Aloes is mentioned 5 times, but this is not the familiar aloe vera we know in America. American aloe is from the Genus, Agave, which is indigenous to the Americas. The Hebrew for aloes is "ahaloth" or "ahalim" while the Greek is the same as English, "aloes." Both terms refer to an oil imported from India distilled from the sandalwood tree, which is also called the lign aloe tree in the *Bible*. (Numbers 24:6)

Adding 5 more for aloes (sandalwood) brings our subtotal to: 307 + 5 = 312 representing nine species.

Mustard Oil

Another source of essential oil in Biblical times was mustard seed, used in medicinal ointments and also as a flavoring. Because of its strength and tendency to burn the skin, mustard oil was always diluted with a neutral base of fat or vegetable oil and used in poultices. It is mentioned 5 times in Jesus' parable of the mustard seed, which is told in Matthew 13, Mark 4; and Luke 13.

In his story, Jesus uses the fact that mustard seeds are among the tiniest of seeds and yet can grow as plants to heights of 12–14 feet—much taller than any other cultivated annual. Mustard stalks grow so tall, in fact, that birds sometimes nest in the tops—a phenomena that can still be witnessed in the Holy land today. What Jesus was trying to say, of course, is that from small spiritual beginnings and a little faith, we can reach great heights and realize great blessings from God.

Adding the five mentions of mustard into the tally we get: 312 + 5 = 317.

Cypress

Cypress leaves and branches were a source of medicinal oil from ancient Egypt as well as throughout Biblical times.

The word cypress is found in the KJV only once—Isaiah 44:14. However, the "oil tree" mentioned in Isaiah 41:19 is thought to have been a reference to cypress also. In Genesis 6:14 Noah is instructed by God to build the ark of gopherwood, which is believed to have been cypress. In I Kings 9:11 what is given as fir in the KJV was actually cypress and is corrected in the NRSV. In Solomon's Song 1:17 the KJV has translated the species as fir, but it was probably cypress, although it could have been pine. With all these considerations, we shall say that cypress has been referenced in the *Bible*, directly or indirectly, five times. 317 + 5 = 322.

Cinnamon, Cumin, and Juniper

Oil of Cinnamon is mentioned 4 times, as is cumin and juniper from which oils were extracted in Biblical times. Cumin seed was also used as a condiment in cooking, and the fragrant branches of juniper were sometimes used to decorate and bring a fresh scent into market booths and dwellings. Adding these three brings our total to: $322 + 12 = 334$.

However, there is more for cinnamon. Both the bark and the leaves of the cinnamon plant produce oil. The oil of the bark is the strongest of the two and the one most familiar to us in the form of cinnamon sticks or ground cinnamon found in spice shelves of modern supermarkets. Cinnamon was one of the ingredients in the holy anointing oil of Exodus 30:22-25. Holy anointing oil is mentioned 65 times in the *Bible* which is tantamount to 65 additional mentions of cinnamon oil.

Taking this into consideration gives us a sum of: $334 + 65 = 399$ references to essential oils with the number of species adding up to 14.

Calamus, Cassia, and Dill

Oils of calamus and cassia are each mentioned 3 times, as is dill. In the case of dill, aromatic oils were extracted from both the plant and the seed. As mentioned earlier in this chapter, dill oil was rubbed on the bodies of gladiators before entering the arena to fight because it reduced anxiety and nervousness. Calamus is also called "aromatic cane" in the NRSV. Cassia is closely related to cinnamon, the two having such similar fragrances that they have been interchanged one for the other. Both may have been considered "oils of gladness," as both have mood elevating effects.

Adding in twelve more mentions for these three we get: $399 + 12 = 411$.

But Calamus and cassia are both ingredients in holy anointing oil, which adds another 65 mentions for each.

Our total now becomes: 411 + 65 (for calamus) + 65 (for cassia) = 541.

Coriander, Henna, Mint, and Pine

Oils of coriander, henna, mint and pine were also used in the Holy Land in ancient times. Henna (NRSV) is called camphire in the KJV. Pine was referred to as an "oil tree" by Biblical people and may have been the tree referred to in Isaiah 41:19, although cypress, fir, or olive would also be legitimate interpretations.

Coriander is an annual plant that produces small, globular, grayish aromatic seeds that were used for flavoring (like caraway or poppy seed) and from which an aromatic oil could be extracted.

Henna is a fragrant flowering shrub or tree common in the Middle East. Its fragrance was extracted for perfumes and cosmetics used by Hebrew women.

The mint of the *Bible* was probably not the familiar peppermint (*Mentha piperita*) or spearmint (*Mentha spicata*) so frequently found in the chewing gums and candies of today. It was probably horse mint (*Mentha longifolia*), which has been grown in the Holy Land for thousands of years. Offerings of mint were often part of the tithe to the temple, where it was used as an air freshener to help cover the smell of blood and burning sacrifices. Biblical mint was also one of the bitter herbs to be eaten with the pascal lamb during the Passover meal. (Exodus 12:8; Numbers 9:11)

These four aromatics (coriander, henna, mint, and pine) are each mentioned twice in the *Bible*. 541 + 8 = 549. We are now up to 21 species.

Roses of the Bible

The Rose of Sharon, immortalized by Solomon in his Song (2:1), and the Rose of Isaiah that will "blossom in the desert" described in Isaiah 35:1, are probably neither one a true rose. The first is probably *Cistus ladanifer* (also known as ladanum or rock rose) and the second

Narcissus tazetta (also known as meadow saffron or cro-cus). Both of these are discussed in Chapter Eight. Both were sources of aromatic oils for medicine or perfume.

The healing capability of cistus or rock rose was noted centuries ago when sheep and goats would accu-mulate the gum of this shrub in their hair as they browsed through the desert. The shepherds noticed that when they rubbed their hands on the wool with this resin, any cuts and scratches would heal much faster. True roses are mentioned in the *Old Testament Apocrypha*. But we won't count those references here. (See Appendix C.)

The Rose of Sharon and the Rose of Isaiah bring our total at this point to: 549 + 2 = 551.

Anise, Bay Leaf, Bdellium, Rue, and Saffron

These six species and sources of essential fragrances are each mentioned once in the *Bible*. The bay tree has always been noted for its aromatic leaves and oils and is a native of the Holy Land. Branches of bay laurel were used to form crowns and head pieces for rulers and vic-torious military leaders of the Roman Empire. Thus, its Latin name: *Laurilus nobilis*.

The word bdellium actually occurs twice (Genesis 2:12 and Numbers 11:7). However in Genesis the Hebrew word "bedolach" translated as "bdellium" in both the KJV and NRSV actually refers to a pearly white mineral, while in Numbers the reference is specifically to an "oily gum." This gum is considered by some scholars to be a distinct species (*Commiphora africana*), closely related to myrrh. However, the general reference to an "oily gum" could also have been frankincense, balm, onycha, galbanum, or a variety of myrrh. All we know for certain is that bdellium was an oily plant known to the wandering children of Israel at the time of their escape from Egypt. In this book we shall tabulate it as a sepa-rate species.

Rue is a strong-smelling perennial Palestinian shrub with gray-green leaves and lemon-yellow clusters of flowers. It was widely used in Biblical times as a condiment, a charm, and as a medicine. It is mentioned as an article for tithing in Luke 11:42.

Saffron was a highly prized aromatic spice used in cooking and medicine. It was imported from India. It is extracted from the aromatic style and stigma of *Crocus sativus.* It is mentioned in the *Bible* in association with spikenard (Song 4:14) as though the two may have been blended as a single ointment.

Adding six more references for these plants brings our total to: 551 + 6 = 557 references to 28 species.

Galbanum and Onycha

Both galbanum and onycha were Biblical medicines. These two oils (pronounced Gal . ba. num and On . i . ca) are explicitly mentioned only once, and both in the same verse (Exodus 30:34). They are both required by God as ingredients in the formula for holy incense. Galbanum (*Ferula gummosa*) is an aromatic, resinous gum related to the giant fennel and was probably imported from Persia or India.

Onycha (*Styrax benzoin*) is another aromatic, resinous gum from the benzoin tree of the Far East. It is also called "benzoin," "friar's balm" and "Java frankincense." Tincture of benzoin was an antiseptic used in hospitals for more than a hundred years, since the mid-1800s. It was the smell most people associated with hospitals.

The ingredients for holy incense are reiterated in the *Old Testament Apocrypha* (Sirach 24:15), including a mention of both galbanum and onycha. But we won't count that in our tally.

There has been some confusion about the identity of onycha among Biblical scholars. Some *Bible* encyclopedias, dictionaries and commentaries say that onycha is "probably a marine shellfish" while others say it was "a sea crab or type of mollusk." The Hebrew word carries such a connotation. However, the term can also refer to the oleo-gum-resin of the aromatic tree of the Far East mentioned above. Since shellfish, crabs (and all fish without scales) are declared unclean and forbidden as food to the Israelites in Deuteronomy 14:9-10, it is unthinkable that they would use such creatures as an ingredient for their holy incense. Besides, the aroma of onycha (the plant) makes a much better perfume than the aroma of onycha (the fish).

Holy incense is mentioned 54 times in the scriptures which is the equivalent of 54 mentions each for galbanum and onycha, plus the one-time mention for each by name. This brings our total to: 557 + 55 (for galbanum) + 55 (for onycha) = 670 references to essential oils in the *Bible,* while our total number of species now stands at 30.

General References to Essential Oils

So far we have only considered oils and aromatic plants that can be identified with particular species. There are numerous references to essential oils whose identity cannot be determined. These include generic references such as odors, perfumes, ointments, and unspecified anointing oils, which always contained essential oils. Every mention of an incense burner (censer) is also a general reference to the use of aromatic oils.

"Spices" is a Biblical term that could refer to either the herbs or to the oils extracted from the herbs. For example, the "spices" used in Jewish burials were always in the form of oils extracted from spicy plant leaves, bark, stems, etc. In either case, whether in solid or liquid form, it is the aromatic or essential oil portion of the spice that is of interest.

The phrase, "sweet savors," as used in the *Bible* was

always a reference to the fragrances of essential oils. However, when the word "savor" was used by itself it usually referred to the pleasant appetizing smell of cooking foods, especially meat. These savors are not included in this tabulation. Only where usage of the word implies essential oils do we include it here.

Citations for these categories of essential oils are found in Appendix A (Table Four-A). They yield the following counts:

Anointing Oils for Kings	61 references
Sweet Savors	50 references
Spices	36 references
Anointing Oils for People	27 references
Incense Censers	20 references
Unspecified Ointments	17 references
Unspecified Incenses	8 references
Odors	7 references
Perfumes	6 references
Oils of Joy	4 references
Essential Oils by Context	4 references

TOTAL GENERAL REFERENCES   240

To this point we have 670 + 240 = 910 Biblical references to essential oils. But we aren't through yet. There are three more species to consider.

Terebinth, Shittah, and Fir

The leaves and twigs of fir trees were an ancient source of essential oil. While the oil of fir is not explicitly mentioned in the *Bible*, fir is mentioned 8 times as lumber and 13 times as a tree. Fir is also one of the possible translations for the "oil tree" mentioned in Isaiah 41:19. Counting this we can add 8 + 13 = 21 bringing the total to 931 and adding another species.

In 21 instances, oak trees cited in the *Bible* (KJV) were true oaks (Genus: Quercus). They were symbols of strength and endurance. True oaks once forested the

Plains of Sharon as well as other areas of the Holy Land. However, there are 12 instances where the KJV has interpreted as "oak" when the actual tree is terebinth (*Pistacia terebinthus*). Terebinth is an aromatic, nut-bearing, oil producing tree with medicinal properties. Terebinth oil is still in use today, mostly in France. The Apocryphal book of Sirach 24:16 calls terebinth the "turpentine tree" because of its strong smelling oil. The *Bible* also refers to terebinth as a "teil tree" in Isaiah 6:13. Terebinth is cited 13 times and brings our running total to: 931 + 13 = 944.

The shittah tree (pronounced <u>sheet</u> . ah) is actually an acacia (*Acacia arabica*), which is an ancient native of the Holy Land and the source of gum arabic. (The word, "shittim," is the plural form of shittah.) Shittah leaves, twigs, and wood are all aromatic sources of oil. The wood contains an essential oil of such strength that it is highly resistant to decay and attack from insects. Being hard and durable, the wood is ideal for cabinet-making. Shittim wood is specified for making carrying poles (Exodus 25:28), for pillars (Exodus 26:32), for tables (Exodus 25:23), and for altars (Exodus 37:25). The Ark of the Covenant was made of Shittim wood. (Exodus 25:10; Deuteronomy 10:3)

The word Shittim is also the name of a Biblical town in Moab, East of the Dead Sea, from whence Joshua sent forth spies. (Joshua 2:1)

There are 26 references to shittim as an aromatic wood or tree. This brings our total references to essential oils and aromatic plants to 944 + 26 = 970 and our total number of species to 33.

Cedar

There is yet one more aromatic to consider before we complete our tally. We have already mentioned cedar-wood several pages back as being specifically referenced six times as an oil, plus four indirect references as an embalming oil. As discussed in Chapter Nine on "The Cedars of Lebanon," the scent of cedarwood was ever-present in the palaces of both King David and King Solomon because they used this wood for construction. There are 25 references to cedar as lumber for building in the *Bible*.

King Solomon also made a point of planting thousands of cedar trees throughout Jerusalem to the extent that "they were as plenteous as the sycamore trees." (II Chronicles 1:15; 9:27) This way the King could not only enjoy the scent of cedar in his palace, but outdoors throughout the capital city as well. So could the residents and visitors of Jerusalem. There are 40 references to living cedar trees in the *Bible*.

This adds another 65 mentions of aromatic oil-producing plants in the *Bible*. Our grand total then becomes 970 + 65 = 1035 references and 33 species.

So What's the Bottom Line?

When the question is posed as to "How many references to essential oils there are in the *Bible*?" you can answer it in several ways. If you followed the logic in completing this tally, you may or may not have agreed with some of the decisions. That's why the thought processes in arriving at these numbers are presented here, so you could decide for yourself. You have several options in answering the question of this chapter:

(1) You could simply cite Table One-A and say, "There are 33 species of essential oils and oil-producing plants mentioned in the *Bible*."

(2) If you want to stick strictly to the specific mentions where particular plant species are named (Table Two-A) , then you can say, "There are 262 references to 33 species of essential oils and the plants that produced them in the *Bible*."

(3) If you want to include the 140 indirect mentions where a specific oil or aromatic plant is clearly implied, but not explicitly stated (Table Three-A), then you can say, "There are 402 references to essential oils and the plants that produced them in the *Bible.*"

(4) If you also include the 240 general mentions where essential oils are clearly implied but their species undetermined (Table Four-A), then you can say, "There are 642 references to essential oils and the plants that produced them in the *Bible.*"

(5) If you also include the fact that many of the 642 *Bible* verses cited in Appendix A refer to more than one specific oil, you can say, "There are 1,035 references to essential oils and the plants that produced them in the *Bible.*"

(6) Another option would be to cite Table Five-A and simply say, "36 of the 39 books of the *Old Testament* (92%) and 10 of the 27 books of the *New Testament* (37%) contain references to essential oils and the plants that produced them."

Say whatever you are comfortable with. The data are all here in this book for you to decide and draw your own conclusions. However, all things considered, you would be on solid ground, both scripturally and intellectually, to state the following, which is our official conclusion for this book:

Essential oils are referenced many times in the *Old and New Testaments*. They were a part of daily living among Israelites, Jews, early Christians, and their Gentile neighbors throughout Biblical times. It would be accurate to say that essential healing oils, their plant sources, and/or their uses are mentioned in the *Bible* more than a thousand times (1,035 to be exact) representing at least 33 species.

Chapter Six
Oils of Joy

In Psalms 45:7 we read the following: "Therefore God, thy God, hath anointed thee with the oil of gladness above thy fellows. All thy garments smell of myrrh, aloes, and cassia out of the Ivory palaces, whereby they have made thee glad."

In Proverbs 27:9 we read: "Ointment and perfume rejoice the heart," where, in Biblical times, ointments and perfumes were either aromatic oils extracted from plants or compounded from them.

In Isaiah 61:1, 3, we read: "The Spirit of the Lord God is upon me, because the Lord hath anointed me; to preach good tidings to the meek, . . to give unto them beauty for ashes, the oil of joy for mourning."

In Hebrews 1:9 we read: "Thou has loved righteousness, and hated iniquity: therefore God, even thy God, hath anointed thee with the oil of gladness."

These four *Bible* passages all have one thing in common. They all refer to anointing oils as vehicles of joy, gladness, and rejoicing. Why would the *Bible* suggest that a physical substance like an oil be associated with an emotional state?

There is a scientific answer to that question. The "oils of joy or gladness" referenced in the scriptures above were all essential oils or vegetable oils containing essential oils. How do we know this? Only essential oils have mood altering properties. Vegetable oils do not. The anointing oils of the *Bible* always contained aromatic essential oils. Essential oils such as frankincense, myrrh, aloes (sandalwood), cassia, and many others are mood elevating. They have emotional impacts that are positive and uplifting. In fact, all essential oils have emotional impacts. This is why.

How Noses are Wired

It all has to do with the way our noses are wired into the brain. The four senses of touch, taste, sight, and hearing are directly connected with the rational part of our cerebral cortex. This means we can think and reason unemotionally when we touch, taste, see, and hear. We can get emotional later if we choose to do so, but these four senses do not directly stimulate our emotions. The intellectual brain is located in the frontal lobes, the mass of neural tissue in your forehead and temples. Whenever you are trying to remember something, you instinctively tap your forehead where the intellectual brain is located. "Jogging our memory," we call it.

Your nose is different. It is wired to the brain backwards to the other four senses. The other four senses pass their signals to the frontal lobes of the brain first and reach the emotional brain second. Smell travels a reverse path. It stimulates emotion first and passes to the rational brain second.

The olfactory nerves connect directly behind the nose to the center of the brain (just above the roof of the mouth) which is the coordinator of our emotions. This region of the brain is variously referred to as the "limbic system," the "diencephalon," or the "amygdala." It involves several organs, including the thalamus, hypothalamus, corpus callosum, fornix, pineal gland, and pituitary gland. We shall call the aggregate of all of these organs the "central brain" or "emotional brain." It includes not only neural cortex but

endocrine glands as well. It functions both electrically and chemically via hormones. We all know from
personal experience that hormones have a great deal
to do with our emotions. So it is not surprising to
learn that the emotional brain secretes hormones
while the intellectual brain does not.

The emotional brain has another interesting property: It does not respond to words that are read, spoken, heard, or felt by braille. It responds to smell.

How the Emotional Brain Works

Think of the central brain as a librarian that files
and catalogues our emotional memories. Our body is
the library. Whenever we experience an emotion, the
central brain takes it in and files it somewhere in your
body. It could be in your heart, your intestines, your
lungs, a specific joint or muscle, or some organ like
the liver or kidneys. In order to recall and access that
memory, the emotional brain (the librarian) has to
locate it in its card index and call it up from wherever it has been stacked in your body. It can then pass
it on to the frontal lobes of your brain where it can be
consciously recalled, revisualized, re-experienced,
and/or articulated.

We store both pleasant and painful memories.
Emotions that we have faced, accepted, and dealt with
are stored as intellectual memories. Such emotions
are resolved and we have grown spiritually through
the experiences that brought them to our awareness.
We can recall such memories in detail, but they do not
control us, give us pain, or make us sick.

Emotions that we have not faced, accepted, nor
dealt with are stored as repressed emotional energy,
waiting for a future time when we can deal with them.
Repressed emotions are unfinished business. They

are lessons unlearned. They are assignments we have not yet chosen to accept. Since they are filed in our bodies in places of which our conscious mind is not aware, they keep us reminded of their existence in a variety of negative ways. They can cause pain, illness, disease, and malfunctions on any and all levels— physical, mental, social, emotional, and spiritual.

This is why essential oils are so valuable in releasing emotional patterns that trouble us, affecting our health and our behavior in ways we do not seem to be able to control. We will not go deeply into this subject here, but there are books and seminars on the topic.

There are two excellent books we shall recommend: *Feelings Buried Alive Never Die* by Karol Truman, and *Releasing Emotional Patterns with Essential Oils* by Carolyn Mein, D.C. Another book, *Molecules of Emotion*, by Candace Pert, Ph.D., is another excellent work that describes the biochemical processes by which our emotions work.

The aromas of essential oils touch our emotions in ways that cannot reach them by any other means. When the roots of our illnesses or conditions stem from buried emotions, essential oils can assist in releasing such blocks to our health and happiness.

The peoples of the *Bible* seemed to understand this and diffused the fragrances of a variety of essential oils in their homes and synagogues and rubbed them on their bodies as well. The Biblical writers may not have understood how aromas feed directly to the emotional brain, but they knew by experience, led by God, that certain perfumes, ointments, and incenses brought joy to their hearts, relieved their stresses, brought them peace and calmness, clarified their thinking, uplifted their spiritual awareness, and assisted them in their prayers, worship, and daily living.

Biblical Oils of Joy

The *Bible* does not tell us what specific oils were in mind when the writers referred to oils of gladness or rejoicing. Psalms 45:7 suggests that among the oils of joy were myrrh, aloes (sandalwood), and cassia. Mint, another Biblical oil, has also been suggested as an oil of gladness, inasmuch as this was the scent often diffused in the Jewish tabernacles along with the holy incense containing galbanum, frankincense, and onycha. The truth is that many oils used in Biblical times were mood elevating.

There is a blend of oils commercially available that has been named Joy™. It contains several uplifting oils in use during Biblical times. These include rosewood, jasmine, roman chamomile, and rose. Joy™ also contains oils not known to be used in Biblical times. These include bergamot, mandarin, lemon, ylang ylang, geranium, and palmarosa.

The term "rose" is mentioned twice in the *Bible* and four times in the Old Testament Apocrypha. It turns out that these six mentions refer to four different species of plants. Only one of them, the one in II Esdras 2:19, is the thorny flowering shrub we recognize as a true rose. In Biblical times, the word "rose" was a name that was applied to many plants with colorful flowers. (See Chapter Eight entitled "Roses of the Scriptures" for more on this.)

As for the rose oil ingredient in the oil of Joy™, it is from the species *Rosa damascena*, a variety related to true roses all over the world, and carries the fragrance we would all recognize and identify as rose. The oil of this flower has the highest electromagnetic frequency of any known substance—320 MHz. It takes 3000-5000 pounds of organic rose petals to produce one pound of rose oil. So it is very precious, indeed, but also a powerful healing oil and especially uplifting spiritually. In fact, in a number of instances throughout history people who have profound spiritual experiences, visions, or miracles report the scent of roses as accompanying the epiphany. In some cultures they say that the fragrance of the rose is the smell of God.

Anoint Yourself With an Oil of Joy

If you have a bottle of Joy™ available to you, try anointing yourself right now as you read this book. It is the first oil we pass around in the *Bible* Oils program outlined in Chapter 14. While the effects of Joy, or any essential oil, is variable and cannot be predicted for any particular individual, many people have found benefit from this particular blend. Some have found it to be an effective mood enhancer. Some have been able to reduce or eliminate their dependence on antidepressant drugs by simply inhaling it, diffusing it in their homes, and/or rubbing it on their bodies.

Take Joy™ or frankincense or sandalwood or myrrh or cassia or cedarwood, which are all "oils of gladness," and put a drop in the palm of your hand. Rub your hands together until they are warm and then gently cup your hands over your mouth and nose (not over your eyes) and breathe. Any excess you can rub on your head or clothing. See what you experience. See how it makes you feel. See if the scriptures were not right when Solomon said, "Ointment and perfume rejoice the heart." (Proverbs 27:9)

It is also worth noting that a state of cheerfulness is elevating to the immune system, helping to protect you from many illnesses. Thus, our emotional state is a key element to our state of health and to the healing of disease. Of course, a positive mental attitude must also be accompanied by right habits of healthful living according to God's laws. But a little oil of joy can go a long way in keeping us well.

> * A NOTE OF CAUTION: If in doing this you get a little oil on the tender skin of your face and it becomes uncomfortably warm, rub on some vegetable oil and the discomfort will go away. Also, the citrus oils of bergamot, mandarin, and lemon found in Joy™ can magnify the effects of ultraviolet and sunlight. So don't apply this oil to your skin and then spend an extended time in sunshine or in a tanning booth during the next twelve hours.

Chapter Seven
The Balm of Gilead

Balm (or balsam) is found seven times in the *Bible* and is one of the very first oils mentioned in Genesis 37:25. (See Appendix A.) From all accounts it was an effective healing ointment for many indications—distilled from the oleo-resin of a tree. In Jeremiah 51:8 it was apparently also an analgesic with pain-relieving capabilities. Also known as the "Balm of Mecca" and the "Balm of Jericho," its principal source is associated with Gilead, which is the country of Jordan, today. The Hebrew meaning of "Gilead" is "rugged," which is an apt description of the mountainous terrain of that land.

The identification and scientific name of the Balm of Gilead has been a matter of debate among Biblical botanists—as is the case for many of the plants of the *Bible.* The authors of the scriptures were more interested in spiritual content than botanical accuracy and often they would use the same word to indicate more than one species.

A variety of specific plants known to have grown in Gilead in that time have been proposed as "the balm" of the *Bible. Balantes aegyptica* (or *Pistacia lentiscus)* is probably the "balm" of Joseph in Genesis 37:25 and 43:11. Scholars draw that conclusion because this particular balm appears to have been of local origin in or near the land of Jacob when Joseph was exiled to Egypt around 1730 B.C. The balm of I Kings 10:10 and Ezekiel 27:17 was probably *Commiphora opobalsamum.* The time frame of this mention of balm would have been after 1000 B.C. Botanically, this balm was in the same family (Burseraceae) as bdellium, frankincense, and myrrh. The Balm of Gilead was a hybrid or cultivar—a species developed by ancient horticulturists. It did not, and could not, grow in the wild. It required the care of a skilled gardener to flourish and survive.

A Visit from the Queen of Sheba

The wealth and wisdom of King Solomon was legendary in his own time. Hearing about the King, Balquis, the Queen of Sheba, decided to visit Jerusalem in 955 B.C. to see for herself the wonders of Solomon's court and to test his wisdom by presenting him with "hard questions." (I Kings 10) Upon arriving with "a very great train of camels bearing spices, gold and precious stones, . . she communed with him of all that was in her heart." Solomon answered all of her questions.

Apparently, Queen Balquis was impressed. "It is a true report that I heard in mine own land of thy acts and of thy wisdom," she said. "Howbeit I believed not the words until I came and mine eyes have seen it: and, behold, the half was not told me: thy wisdom and prosperity exceedeth the fame which I heard."

As she departed to return to the land of Sheba in southern Arabia, she left Solomon with considerable gifts, including 120 talents of gold, precious stones, spices, and balm.

Tradition has it that Solomon was so impressed with the fragrance and healing properties of the balm oil that he persuaded the Queen to send him some seeds and young trees by which he established a grove near Jericho. Thus, the Balm of Gilead acquired another name—the "Balm of Jericho."

Theophrastes, a Greek writer of around 300 B.C., mentions two groves of balm trees in the holy land present in his time, including the one at Jericho planted by Solomon. In Theophrastes' time a pound of balm oil sold for two pounds of silver, which would be about $150 in today's market. The oil was described as "yellow, tenacious, and sticking to the fingers" When a few drops were rubbed into a wound, it was said to bring about rapid healing. A few drops taken internally or applied on the belly were said to "strengthen a weakened stomach" and was "the best stomachic known."

Leaf Like Rue; Fruit Like Terebinth

Theophrastes described the balm tree as follows: "The tree is as tall as a good sized pomegranate and is much branched. It has a leaf like rue, but it is pale. It is evergreen. The fruit is like that of the terebinth in size and color, and this, too, is very fragrant, indeed, even more so than the gum."

The balm trees of Jericho were still there in Roman times. In 35 B.C. the Egyptian Queen, Cleopatra, acquired rights to the groves in the Holy Land with the help of Mark Anthony, then a ruler of Rome.

Herod I ("The Great") was a Roman governor of Galilee who pleased the Roman Senate because of his success in subduing Galilean bandits, ruling with an iron hand and with total loyalty to Rome. He was about twenty-five years of age when the Senate rewarded him by giving him a prize that still required conquest. The prize was Jerusalem and the Holy Land. His new title was to be "King of the Jews."

In order to take Jerusalem and seize power over his prize, he had to dethrone the Judean ruler, Antigonus II, who was an enemy of Rome. This he did with the help and military forces of Mark Anthony in 35 B.C. In return for the assistance of Mark Anthony, Herod agreed to send the revenues from the sales of balm to Cleopatra in an annual lump sum of cash. (Shall we say that Anthony and Cleopatra were very good "friends" and were "seriously dating" at the time.)

Cleopatra Cashes In

Anthony's gift to Cleopatra was no small one. From her Palestinian groves she collected 200 talents a year. Since one talent was equal to 3,600 shekels, her profit from the balm would be 720,000 shekels a year. In that day, this bit of extra income could buy 103,000 tons of grain, 48,000 oxen, 4,800 horses, or 1,200 chariots.

Thus one can begin to appreciate just how valuable this essential oil actually was and how potent its healing powers must have been to generate such income. Cold coinage cannot directly heal nor maintain the most precious commodity a person can possess—which is health. But aromatic oils can, did, and do promote healing, health, and longevity, awakening God's healing grace within our bodies.

The cultivated balm groves of Biblical times are known to have survived at least until the seventh century A.D. when the Holy Land was overrun by Moslem invaders. By the Christian Crusades of the eleventh century, the groves had all disappeared without a trace. A living resource that had produced healing oils for more than 1,500 years had been destroyed never to grow again in the Holy Land.

Jesus and the Last Grove

The world's last grove of surviving balm trees was by the Well of Matarya, near Cairo in Egypt. It was planted by Cleopatra around 35 B.C. This has always been considered by Christians to be the place that Mary and Joseph stayed when they fled to Egypt with Baby Jesus. The story is told in Matthew 2:1-23.

The same King Herod that Mark Anthony had helped take control of the throne in Jerusalem was still ruler when Jesus was born. When the wise men came seeking "he who is born King of the Jews," Herod became alarmed that the newborn child, fore-told by the wise men, might be a future threat to his throne. The title, "King of the Jews," had been for-mally bestowed on him by Rome, and he was not will-ing to take any chances of losing either the title or the territory.

Slaughter of the Innocents

When Herod conceived a plan to kill all of the baby boys in Bethlehem who were two years of age or under, Joseph was warned by God in a dream to take his wife and son and flee to Egypt, which he did. The Holy Family was instructed to remain there until they received a sign to return.

When Herod died a couple of years later, God appeared to Joseph in a dream again and told him that it would be safe to return to Israel. It was then that the Holy Family came and settled in a Galilean village called Nazareth in the neighborhood of where Mary had grown up as a child, near the home of her parents and kin.

During those two years near Cairo, infant Jesus and his parents would have seen Cleopatra's grove of balm trees many times. Mary and Joseph with the Babe no doubt walked beneath their branches, enjoyed their fragrance, and sat in their shade. Some of the oil from those trees, distilled nearby, may have been used by Mary and Joseph

For more than 1,600 years, Christian pilgrims visiting the Well of Matarya could see living trees that had sheltered Jesus, Mary and Joseph. But, alas, the last one died 400 years ago, in the seventeenth century, leaving no heirs and no offspring.

Thus the Balm of Gilead that had blessed the Biblical peoples of Egypt, Arabia, and the Holy Land for thousands of years became extinct—its healing oil no longer available—lost forever in the Dark Ages of Medieval history.

Chapter Eight
Roses of the Holy Land

As we have mentioned before, Biblical writers were not botanists. They were not particularly concerned about precise identifications of the blossoming plants with which they flowered their poesy and prose. The term translated as "rose" in the *Bible* was a word of particularly imprecise usage. It was applied to a variety of colorful blooms grown wild or cultivated in the Holy Land. Today there are over 5,000 varieties of true roses that have been named and scientifically identified.

Flowers identified as some form of a rose have been mentioned as far back as the Ayurvedas of India dating 5,000 B.C. Roses were praised by the Greek writer, Homer, in the Iliad where Aphrodite anoints the body of Hector with rose oil. Homer lived in the 9th century B.C., at about the same time as King Solomon and the Queen of Sheba. Rose-scented ointments have been produced in the Middle East by maceration in various fatty oils for thousands of years. Rose water is also an ancient Middle Eastern product. where rose petals are soaked in water, the petals strained out, and more petals put in to concentrate the resulting perfume.

Distilling the oil from rose petals with steam was an art known to ancient Arabians and Egyptians as far back as 5000 B.C. However, distillation was a technology lost to the Western World with the fall of Rome in 500 A.D. It was not rediscovered until 400 years later by Arabians.

I Am the Rose of Sharon

When King Solomon sang, "I am the Rose of Sharon and the Lily of the Valleys . . ." (Song of Solomon 2:1) the most likely candidates he had in mind were probably a bright red tulip-like flower (*Tulpa montana*) or the sweet fragrant gum-bearing rock rose (*Cistus ladanifer*)—both of which flourished in the Plains of Sharon.

The myrrh mentioned in Genesis 37:25 and 45:11 may also have been cistus or rock rose, and not true myrrh (*Commiphora myrrha*). Scholars conclude this because the Midianites carrying "myrrh" in Genesis had passed through the regions of Gilead and Sharon going south toward Egypt, which would have been the wrong direction for myrrh to be transported. Myrrh does not come from north of Jacob's location, but from the south next to Egypt. Rock rose was a similar gum-bearing plant whose oil may have been confused for myrrh and, perhaps, substituted for it.

The Desert Shall Blossom as the Rose

When Isaiah prophesied that "the desert shall rejoice and blossom as the rose," (KJV) he was probably thinking of a plant of the lily family, a crocus (NRSV) whose technical name was *Narcissus tazetta*. This flower was also known as the meadow saffron and narcissus.

These are the only two references to a rose in the *Bible* and both are in the *Old Testament*. However there are five mentions of roses in the *Old Testament Apocrypha*—books of Jewish history and wisdom that fill the gap between Malachi and Matthew. While some Christians accept these as legitimate scriptures, some do not. (See Appendix B.) In any case, they do provide an accurate account of the beliefs and customs of the people of the Holy Land in the centuries just before the coming of Jesus.

The Rose of Jericho

In the Apocryphal book called "The Wisdom of Solomon," we read: "Let us crown ourselves with rose buds before they be withered." (Wisdom 2:8)

In the book of Sirach (also called Ecclesiasticus) we have three verses referring to roses: "Hearken unto me, ye holy children, and bud forth as a rose growing by the brook of the field." (Sirach 39:13)

"As the flower of roses in the spring of the year, as lilies by the rivers of waters, as branches of the frankincense tree in the time of summer." (Sirach 50:8)

"I grew tall like a palm tree in Engedi, and like rose plants in Jericho." (Sirach 24:14)

In these three cases, authorities believe the rose that is indicated was actually a tall bushy shrub known as rose laurel or oleander, Nerium oleander. Rose Laurel is not a true rose at all like the thorny shrubs we know. These colorful pink flowering evergreen bushes grow ten to twelve feet high and can be found blooming in the wilderness and lining the banks of the river Jordan still today.

Roses of the Mountains

In the Apocryphal book of Second Esdras we read about "seven mighty mountains on which roses and lilies grow." (II Esdras 2:19) These mountains would have been in present-day Lebanon, Syria, or Turkey. In this scripture, we are talking about true roses— either the Phoenician Rose (Rosa phoenicia) or the Rose of Damascus (Rosa damascena) or both. Both grew wild and both were also cultivated. Both were called the "rose of the mountains." It is these latter species that contain the most oil and from which the

Middle Eastern rose perfume industry has sprung since the tenth century A.D.

The land of Phoenicia was called Tyre in the *Bible* and was well established in international trade at least as far back as 1400 B.C. Tyre is mentioned 58 times in the *Bible*—46 times in the *Old Testament* and 12 times in the *New Testament*. King Hiram of Tyre established trade with the Israelites during the reigns of David and Solomon and helped Solomon build his temple. (II Samuel 5, 24; I Kings 5, 7, 9; I Chronicles 14, 27; II Chronicles 2) Rose oil and other rose products were manufactured in Tyre and traded throughout the Mediterranean civilizations, from Jerusalem to Egypt, to Cypress, to Rome, and to the land we now call Spain.

The Roses of Phoenicia and Damascus are both ancient species that date back to the beginnings of recorded history. Rose oil was popular with the Romans, Arabians, Egyptians, and Greeks of Biblical times. Although not mentioned in the *Bible*, the essential oil of the rose was no doubt used by the Hebrews of the *Old Testament* as well as the Christians of the *New Testament*. It was definitely a part of the cultures of the Holy Land and surrounding countries.

Too Expensive to be Widely Used

Rose oil may not have been popular among the Jews and early Christians because of its cost, which was more than for any other oil, including frankincense, myrrh, and balm. As stated earlier in Chapter Six, it takes 3,000-5,000 pounds of rose petals to produce one pound of rose oil, which makes it one of the most expensive oils in the world. However, its healing characteristics are outstanding. known for its benefits on all levels, body, mind, and spirit. It's electromagnetic frequency of 320 MHz is the highest known of all oils. It is one of the constituents of the oil of Joy mentioned in Chapter Six of this book.

Summary of Scriptural References to Rose

In summary, we find that there are two references to rose in the *King James Version* of the *Bible*, neither of which are actually true roses:

• The Rose of Isaiah was a colorful tulip-like flower (*Tulpa montana*) also called Meadow Saffron, Crocus, and Narcissus.

• The Rose of Sharon (in the Song of Solomon) is thought to be cistus or ladanum (*Cistus ladanifer*), which was also called Rock Rose.

• We find five more scriptural references to roses in the *Old Testament Apocrypha*, only one of which is a true rose.

• Four of the references (three in Sirach and one in Wisdom) are to the oleander bush (*Nerium oleander*) which was called by several names including Jericho Rose, Rose Laurel, Bay Rose and Rose of the Brook.

• The one and only scriptural reference to a true rose (*Rosa damascena* or *Rosa phoenicia*) is found in II Esdras 2:19. These two species of true roses are also called Roses of the Mountains.

Chapter Nine
The Cedars of Lebanon

The temples and palaces of King David and King Solomon were built of cedar as described in the books of Samuel, Kings, and Chronicles. "And Hiram, King of Tyre. sent messengers to David and cedar trees and carpenters and masons: and they built David a house." (II Samuel 5:11) When David died, Solomon became king and set about to build a temple to God. He made a proposal to Hiram, the King of Tyre (Phoenicia), to "hew cedar trees out of Lebanon." (I Kings 5:6) King Hiram's end of the bargain was to supply all the building materials that Solomon would request. This included not only cedar, but fir, cypress, and hewn stones.

Hiram agreed to Solomon's proposal with these words,

> "I will do all thy desire concerning timber of cedar. . . My servants shall bring them down from Lebanon unto the sea; and I will convey them by sea in floats unto the place that thou shalt appoint me, and will cause them to be discharged there, and thou shalt receive them: and thou shalt accomplish my desire, in giving food for my household. So King Hiram gave Solomon cedar trees. . . according to all his desire." (I Kings 5:8-10)

So Solomon "built the house, and finished it; and covered the house with beams and boards of cedar." (I Kings 6:9) "And he built the walls of the house within with boards of cedar, both the floor of the house, and the walls of the ceiling." (I Kings 6:15)

What Hiram was to receive in return was 20,000 cors of wheat and 20 cors of fine oil every year for as long as it took to complete the temple. (I Kings 5:11) In addition, there would be a peace agreement between the two nations.

Israel's Price for Solomon's Temple

To get an idea of Solomon's cost in this endeavor, consider that a cor is 14 bushels (the maximum load a donkey could carry). In liquid units this was approximately 60 gallons. Hence, Solomon's cost to tap into the resources of Tyre and Lebanon (a province of Tyre) was 20,000 donkey loads of grain (280,000 bushels) and 1,200 gallons of oil. That's a lot of oil.

Most of this oil was probably of a type used for food or burning in lamps (probably olive, although some of it could have been almond, walnut, linseed, pistachio, or sesame). Some of it was probably essential and aromatic.

The Hebrew word that appears in the original text is "shemen," which can be translated with equal validity as "oil" or as "ointment." For example, the Hebrew word "shemen" was translated as "ointment" in fourteen Bible passages: II Kings 20:13; Psalms 133:2; Proverbs 27:9, 16; Ecclesiastes 7:1; 9:8; 10:1; Song of Solomon 1:3a, 3b; 4:10; Isaiah 1:6; 39:2; 57:9; and Amos 6:6. Ointments were always compounds of essential oils. Therefore, we can safely conclude that some of the oils Solomon sent were essential.

Any way you interpret it, King Hiram was well compensated for the resources taken from his land, but the land, itself, received no compensation. It was totally pillaged and robbed.

The Trees of the Lord

In King David's day, when he wrote Psalms 104:16, "The cedars of Lebanon" were considered to be "the Trees of the Lord, that He planted." According to reports during David's reign, the cedars of Lebanon were magnificent, indeed, attaining towering heights and great diameters. They lived to a great age, some exceeding as many as 2,000 years. Some of the trees alive in David's day would have been still living at the time of Jesus, while a few cedars that were seedlings in Christ's day may yet be alive today, hidden away in the rugged mountains of Lebanon—ancient giants, survivors of an era long past.

Although small patches and remnants of cedar remain in the remotest reaches of Lebanon's rugged terrain, the vast forests of Solomon's days are no more. Today, the cedars of Lebanon (*Cedrus libani*) are an endangered and protected species no longer available for their lumber nor for their essential oil.

Today we extract cedarwood oil from *Cedrus atlanticus*, a species most similar to the Biblical cedars and which are found in the Atlas Mountains of Greece, as well as parts of Morroco and Algeria.

The Egyptians Did it First

The massive and majestic stands of cedar that once forested the peaks and valleys of Lebanon were first exploited by the Egyptian Pharaohs. They used the aromatic and durable timber for temples and dwellings. The wood was also used to make musical instruments, coffins, and boats. This was over a span of many centuries before, during, and after the days of Moses. Egypt's impact on the supply was negligible enough that the forests were still plentiful centuries later when Solomon set his mind on a palace and a tabernacle of cedarwood.

The idea of a cedar dwelling for a king, as well as a place for worship, is an excellent application of the power of essential oils. Cedar is a fragrant wood, due to its oil content, whose aroma lasts indefinitely. A building made of cedarwood would always carry the faint scent of cedar oil. Hence, any Biblical reference to using cedarwood as a building material is an indirect reference to the application of an essential oil. The *Old Testament* contains 25 mentions of cedarwood as a building material and 40 mentions of cedar as trees or timber.

Cedarwood: Cure for Senility and Alzheimers?

It turns out that inhaling the oil of cedarwood increases the ability to think clearly and enhances the awareness needed for effective prayer and meditation. This is because, of all the essential oils of the world, cedarwood contains the highest concentration of sesquiterpenes (98%). The sesquiterpenes in cedarwood have the ability to pass through the blood-brain barrier and oxygenate the brain directly upon inhalation by way of the nasal passages and the olfactory nerves. It has even been suggested that cedarwood oil might prevent senility and Alzheimer's disease.

While the biochemistry of the process just described was not known in ancient times, the fact that cedarwood created an environment that enhanced clear thinking was appreciated by the Egyptians. They were, perhaps, the first civilization to distill cedarwood oil, something they had been doing as far back as 3500 B.C. They used the oil for a variety of purposes, including temple worship, emotional clearing, embalming, enhancing mental clarity, and as an insect repellent. No doubt some of these facts were also appreciated by the Israelites as well, who learned the art of creating and applying essential oils during their Egyptian captivity.

It is probably no coincidence that both David and

Solomon chose cedar as the wood for their homes and temples. For a king, who has to make decisions every day that affect thousands of subjects, living in an environment where they would inhale cedarwood oil every day would contribute toward wise judgments and help keep their consciousness elevated on a spiritual level. Perhaps the wisdom of Solomon was even greater than we thought and included a sophisticated knowledge of essential oils and how they could assist him in ruling his kingdom in an effective way pleasing to God.

Environmental Forestry

Unfortunately, Solomon's wisdom did not extend to a sense of responsibility to the environment nor an awareness of the irreversible destruction his insatiable desire for cedar timber would have on the Lebanese landscape. Singlehandedly, he practically brought to extinction a hallowed species of one of God's most sacred creations.

The scale of his exploitation was staggering. King Solomon conscripted 30,000 Israelite men to harvest the trees and transport the timber to Jerusalem. They were sent to Lebanon in shifts of 10,000 men each for one month, then two months back home, then back to Lebanon again and again the year round, until the work was completed. They were assisted by 150,000 slaves who not only cut the trees, but also quarried great stones to be laid as the foundations and pillars of the temple. To manage and administrate such an ambitious undertaking, there were 3,300 supervisors. The total work force came to 183,000 men, working day in and day out for years, methodically stripping the lush forestlands of Lebanon of their centuried treasures, destroying them forever. (I Kings 5:13-15)

Solomon had no idea of the damage he was doing by such a massive assault, and he knew nothing of conservation. Seven years they labored on the temple "for the glory of God" and yet another thirteen on a private palace. Solomon's home became known as the "House of the Forest of Lebanon." It was this edifice that so impressed the Queen of Sheba during her visit in 955 B.C.

First the Axes, Then the Goats

The decimated forests would have recovered if nature would have been allowed to take her course. Instead, goats were allowed to browse off the new young growth that would have eventually become a great forest again. Goats are thorough foragers, stripping the fertile hillsides of their cover such that the wind and rain eroded away the rich top soil that had accumulated there for eons. With the irreplaceable resource of soil removed, the cedars could no longer take root and re-establish themselves. What had been a good land of bubbling brooks and copious springs flowing out of the valleys and hills, was left to become one of the most desolate and impoverished in all the world.

We must give Solomon some credit for conservation, however. While he demolished the cedar forests of Lebanon, he did his part to preserve the species. He planted thousands of Lebanese cedar trees all over Jerusalem, whose subsequent generations still grace that city today. (II Chronicles 1:15; 9:27) Thus, the fragrant oils of the cedar tree were wafted throughout the city in Solomon's day, another natural application of aromatherapy, like the Garden of Eden.

This was not exactly a reforestation program that benefitted Lebanon in any way. Furthermore, the

Jerusalem climate and environment never produced cedars of the majesty and scale that once reigned over the hills of Lebanon.

Restoring a Legacy

The distinctive pyramidal image of the tree adorns the flag of Lebanon today. Fortunately, in addition to the protection the government affords, there is a Christian sect, the Patriarch of Maronites, who manage the remnants of cedar groves that remain. The Maronites have initiated a long-term replanting program in an attempt to reforest the once verdant hills of that Biblical land.

It will take a thousand years of such care and effort to restore even a portion of the timbered glory that was once the pride of the ancient world.

Chapter Ten
Myrrh: The Most Popular Oil of the Bible

Myrrh is referenced more than any other aromatic oil of the *Bible*. It is the first to be mentioned (Genesis 37:25) and the last (along with Frankincense) in Revelation 18:13. As the word "mor" in Hebrew, it is used twelve times. Its perfume was praised by Solomon eight times in his song of love. (Song of Solomon 1:13; 3:6; 4:6, 14: 5:1, 5a, 5b, 13) It was required by God in his formula for holy anointing oil given to Moses in Exodus 30:23. Esther bathed in myrrh for six months in preparation for her marriage to the king. (Esther 2:12) David sings of myrrh as an oil of gladness in Psalms 45. While in Proverbs 7:17 Solomon warns of the temptress who perfumes her bed with myrrh.

The sweet spice of "stacte" is an oil mandated by the Lord in compounding holy incense for the tabernacle in Exodus 30:34; stacte is another name for myrrh. Bdellium, an oily gum mentioned in Numbers 11:7, may also have been a variety of myrrh, but we won't count it as myrrh in this book.

These verses, alone, would add up to fifteen *Old Testament* references to the oil of myrrh, but there are more—many more. The anointing oil of Exodus 39:23 is mentioned 65 times, and the holy incense of Exodus 30:34, which also contained myrrh, is referenced 54 times. Table Two-A in Appendix A reveals four more indirect references to myrrh in Genesis in the form of embalming spices and another citation (Exodus 25:6) indicates myrrh as an ingredient for holy fragrances. Adding up what we have to this point brings us to a figure of 139 references to myrrh in the *Old Testament*, alone. But there are more in the *New Testament* besides the one in Revelation already mentioned.

Mor is Hebrew for myrrh, which is the language of the *Old Testament*. But the original *New Testament* was written in Greek. The Greek words for myrrh are several: Smurna, Smurnizo and Muron.

The First and the Last

When Matthew tells the story of the three wise men, he chose the word "smurna" for myrrh. (Matthew 2:11) Thus, when presented to him at his birth, myrrh was one of the very first oils Jesus would receive in his life time on earth. It was also one of the last.

When Jesus was about to be nailed to the cross at Golgotha, he was offered wine mixed with myrrh—a common practice at the time. The Romans thought that adding a little myrrh to wine would make it less inebriating and less likely to produce drunkenness. They also claimed that drinking myrrh in wine would alleviate arthritis. The choice of Greek by Mark to tell the story was "Smurnizo." (Mark 15:23)

When Joseph of Arimathea and Nicodemus came to prepare the body of Christ for burial (John 19:39), they brought oils of sandalwood (aloes) and myrrh (smurna)—a large quantity (100 litras or 75–100 pounds). In today's retail market that would be $150,000–$200,000 worth of essential oils. This tells us two things: (1) Joseph and Nicodemus were very wealthy; and (2) Their regard and reverence for their Lord and redeemer was very great, indeed.

Thus, not only is myrrh a topic of both the first and last books of the *Bible*, it was also an oil offered to Christ at both the beginning and the end of his life.

Adding in the four references to myrrh in Matthew, Mark, John, and Revelation to our *Old Testament* total of 139 brings us to 143 Biblical mentions of myrrh. But we aren't through yet. There are still more.

The myrrh offered to Jesus in the wine at his crucifixion and in the burial spice for his body after death may not have been the only times myrrh played a role in the last days of his ministry on earth.

The Mystery of the Anointing Woman

All four Gospels tell a story of a woman who anoints Jesus with a very costly ointment, but the four versions do not all agree as to when, where, who, what, how, and why? In telling this story, the Gospels pose for us six questions or puzzles to solve as follows:

1. When did it happen?
2. Where did it happen?
3. Who was the woman?
4. What was the ointment?
5. How was it applied?
6. And why was the story told?

In other words, question number six asks, "What is the spiritual lesson to be gleaned from the narrative?" because the Gospel writers all had a philosophical, theological, or moral point in mind with every story they chose to include in their accounts of the life of Jesus. In fact, the focus of the *Bible* writers on the spiritual message caused them to be less than perfect in their attention to geographical, historical, and material detail. This is the main reason it is difficult to construct a book on essential oils (such as this) from a source (like the *Bible*) whose theme was religion—not the properties of plants and their uses.

Origin of the Four Gospels

The four Gospel accounts of Jesus and the woman with the perfumed ointment are told in Matthew 26:1-13; Mark 14:1-9; Luke 7:36-50, and John 11:1-2; 12:1-8. It is important to understand how and in what order these Gospels were written. Because he was the most educated of the Twelve Disciples, Matthew was appointed to keep notes on Jesus' life and sayings, which he recorded in Aramaic. Years later, when Matthew enlarged his notes into a Gospel, he wrote in Greek, the universal language of the day. Mark and Luke both had access to Matthew's notes, which is why the first three Gospels correspond so closely in word and detail.

Mark's Gospel is the shortest and was probably the first to be completed (between 60 and 68 A.D.) followed by Matthew and Luke (c. 65-80 A.D.). Mark was not one of the Twelve and did not have the opportunity to be a firsthand witness to much that his Gospel contains. Besides Matthew as a source, Mark's Gospel also relied on information obtained from Barnabas, his uncle, and from Peter, with whom he traveled after Jesus' death and ressurection. Neither was Luke one of the Twelve. Thus, the first three Gospels were derived principally from Matthew's notes. John's Gospel was the last to be published—sometime between 80 and 90 A.D. He would have been familiar with the other three accounts but did not copy any of them literally, relying mostly on his own notes and memories.

With respect to the six questions posed, here is how each Gospel answers them:

(1) WHEN? Matthew and Mark say "two days before the passover" when Jesus shall be betrayed. Luke does not say when exactly, except that he tells the story as if it occurred near the beginning of Jesus' ministry, perhaps 2-3 years before his crucifixion. John places the event during Jesus' last week, as did Matthew and

Mark, but "six days before the passover." So we have three possible times.

(2) WHERE? Luke's location for the story is not mentioned except as being near a "city" and, hence, is unknown. The other three writers all place the incident in Bethany, except that Matthew and Mark say it occurred in the "house of Simon the Leper," while John says it was in the "house of Lazarus whom Jesus had raised from the dead." While the town is not given by Luke, he places it in the House of "Simon the Pharisee," with no mention of whether he was also a leper. So we have three possible locations.

(3) WHO? Matthew and Mark merely refer to "a woman" with no clue as to her name, place of origin, personal characteristics, or relationship to Jesus. Luke calls her "a woman from the city" but does not identify her. Instead, he elaborates on the point that "she was a sinner," implying that she was probably a harlot. John is the only one to give the woman a name and emphatically insists, almost as if he needed to correct the other three writers (especially Luke), that the woman was Mary, the sister of Martha and Lazarus. So here, again, we have three possible candidates for the woman.

(4) WHAT? This question has to do with what was contained in the ointment? The Greek word chosen in telling the story used by all the Gospel writers is "muron." The word was used 13 times: 3x by Matthew, 2x by Mark, 4x by Luke, and 4x by John. Muron is a Greek word for myrrh, but was also used as a more general designation for any variety of ointment or perfume.

This was because myrrh was used as a fixing oil in most aromatic preparations. In the fragrance business, a fixative is an oil that, when mixed with other oils, will "fix" the odors, causing the fragrances to last longer. Myrrh is one of the most effective fixing oils of all and has been used for thousands of years throughout the world. The ancient cultures of China, India, Sumer,

Babylon, Arabia, Persia, Phoenicia, and Egypt all used myrrh for this purpose, as did the Israelites, Jews, Greeks, Romans, early Christians, and perfumers of every century to the present.

It is interesting to note that myrrh is the only oil mandated by God to be an ingredient in both the holy anointing oil and the holy incense. (Exodus 30:23, 34) Apparently God was a knowledgeable aromatherapist who understood the basic principles of blending fragrances to always include a fixative.

You May Have Worn Myrrh And Didn't Know It

Myrrh is a fixative in many contemporary perfumes and colognes today. You may recognize or have used some of them. Among feminine fragrances they include the following: Fidji® (Laroche), Givenchy III® (Givenchy), Alliage® (Estee Lauder), Ravissa® (Maurer & Wirtz, and LeSport® (St. Laurent)—which also contains Sandalwood (aloes).

Myrrh is also used in these modern men's fragrances: Vetiver® (Carmen), Matchbelli® (Matchbelli), and Punjab® (Capucci).

But back to the question of "What was in the ointment used by the woman?" The thirteen uses of the Greek "muron" in the four Gospels are all translated as "ointment." in both the *Authorized King James Version* (KJV) and the *New Revised Standard Version* (NRSV) except in John where the NRSV uses the term "perfume." The *New International Version* (NIV) also translates muron as "perfume."

So why did the translators all choose to use generic definitions of the Greek "muron" when they could just as well have chosen to translate the word as "myrrh?" Evidently none of the translators were knowledgeable in the art of perfumery or aromatherapy. They did not realize that myrrh was a fixative in almost every ointment of that time. The use of myrrh for fixing was so universal that the word "muron," that had originally meant "myrrh," had become synonymous with "ointment" or "perfume." Regardless of how the *Bible* translators interpreted the word, what we know for certain is that when the word "muron" was used, myrrh was definitely an ingredient in the mixture. (It is interesting to note that when muron was used in Revelation 18:13, it was translated as "ointment" in the KJV, but changed to myrrh in the NRSV.)

So It Contained Myrrh . . But What Else?

In answering the question of what was in the ointment, let's start by saying it was myrrh in all four Gospels. At last they all agree on something! Adding these 13 references to the 143 we already have brings the total Biblical mentions for myrrh to 156.

What about spikenard? Matthew and Luke do not mention another oil except muron or myrrh. But in Mark and John, they refer to an "ointment of nard or spikenard." In these two Gospels the Greek uses "muron" in association with "nardos pistikos" where nardos means "nard or spikenard" and pistikos means "genuine or pure." Furthermore, Matthew, Mark, and Luke all describe the woman's container as an "alabaster box."

Spikenard is an aromatic flowering herb native to the Himalayan Mountains of India and Tibet. In Biblical times it was imported from there to the Holy Land and shipped in boxes carved from alabaster. This fact is yet another clue that the woman's ointment contained spikenard. In ancient times the term alabaster referred to a type of marble —a metamorphosed calcium carbonate. In modern times, the word is also used to designate a dense form of gypsum (hydrated calcium sulphate) as well as some forms of travertine or cave rock. The

Sanskrit root of the Greek and Latin word for alabaster is another clue that ties the reference to India and spikenard.

So we see that all four Gospels either refer to spikenard directly (Mark and John) and/or refer to spikenard indirectly by reference to an alabaster box (Matthew, Mark, and Luke).

That makes it unanimous among the Gospels on both counts. The oil used by the woman was a blend of spikenard with myrrh.

How Precious?

Before we go on to the next question (5), let's comment on the fact that in all four Gospels the "ointment" is "precious" and/or "very costly." John mentions a quantity of "one litra" which is a Greek unit equal to 12-16 English ounces. The KJV translates it as "a pound." The prices of myrrh and spikenard are both pretty high, with spikenard being, perhaps, a bit more costly than myrrh. In twenty-first century American dollars, the retail cost of a pound of spikenard mixed with myrrh would be in the range of $1500 to $2000. For common laborers in that time and place, that amount of money would have been a year's wages.

(5) HOW? The question is "How and where was the oil applied?" Matthew says, "she poured it on his head." Mark also says, "she poured it on his head," but prior to that he states that, "she brake the box (KJV) or "broke open the jar" (NRSV). The breaking here does not mean a literal breaking of the alabaster container, but breaking a thick waxy layer that customarily sealed the precious contents from leakage or exposure to air. So at this point we have two accounts that say Jesus was anointed on his head.

Luke and John disagree. Both of these writers say that Jesus was anointed on his feet and that the woman wiped them with her hair. So here we have a 50:50 split on how the oil was applied.

An Omen of Imminent Death

(6) WHY? The question is "Why was this story included in the Gospel? What was its point?"

Matthew, Mark, and John all agree that the oil was applied as a symbolic preparation for Jesus' imminent death, which in John was six days away, while in Matthew and Mark it was only two days away. This also gives more credibility to the idea of myrrh constituting a significant part of the ointment, inasmuch as myrrh was a customary burial oil, while spikenard was not. The unexpected anointment with a burial ointment by an uninvited stranger at one of Jesus' last meals was tantamount to an omen of his physical demise soon to come—a fact that had not yet been grasped, accepted, nor understood by his closest disciples at that point in time.

Although Jesus had told them of his fatal destiny in Jerusalem on several occasions, the twelve disciples were still in denial over the matter when the woman poured the oil over their master.

A Setting for a Parable

In Luke, the incident is set a couple of years before Jesus' final week in Jerusalem. Luke's purpose in telling the story is to provide an illustration of Jesus parable of the two debtors (one who owed a little and one who owed a lot). As the parable goes, both debtors were forgiven of their debts, but the one forgiven of the greater debt held the greater gratitude toward the generous creditor who had released him. The analogy created by the story is the difference between Simon the Pharisee (who had always lived a life of righteousness incurring only a small debt of sin) compared to the prostitute (who had lived a life of great sin). Jesus noted that the pious Simon had not anointed him with oil (which was a customary courtesy toward guests of honor) nor had he expressed his love and devotion in recognition of Jesus as a redeemer and forgiver of sin. By contrast, the poor distraught woman continuously wept and expressed her devotion to Jesus without ceasing. Jesus forgave her of her sins, as he did those of Simon, but the greater gratitude and appreciation was from the woman, having been released from the greater debt.

So with respect to why the story was told, we have three Gospels for the burial symbology and one for a parable on forgiveness and gratitude. But there is yet another reason the story has been included in the scriptures.

In Matthew and Mark "some of the disciples" (not just one) objected to the consumption of such a costly amount of oil, saying it could have been sold and the money given to the poor. In Luke, no one is reported as objecting to the pouring out of the expensive oil. In John, it is specifically Judas, and no one else, who objects. John suggests that Judas may have been interested in the money the oil could bring for selfish reasons. In all cases, Jesus reproved the disapproving disciples saying that the woman had done a good and proper thing and would be well remembered in history for her act of repentance, sacrifice, and devotion.

Solving the Mystery of the Anointing Woman

To this point we have presented the four Gospel versions of this story and have noted their differences and apparent contradictions. The only place a unanimous agreement was found between the four was in the content of the ointment, which had to be both myrrh and spikenard. This brings our tally for scriptural mentions of myrrh to 143 + 13 = 156. That

makes myrrh, by far, the most mentioned oil of the
Bible with frankincense in second place with a score
of 81. (See Appendix A.)

What about all the discrepancies between these
four accounts? Are these really contradictions of
scripture? Or is there an explanation that makes
them all true? Here is how we resolve them.

Three Women, Three Times, Three Places

Luke's version is set near an un-named city in the
first year or two of Jesus' ministry. The other three are
set in Bethany during Holy Week, 2-6 days before
Jesus died. Luke's account is parallel with John's in
that a woman anointed Jesus' feet and dried them
with her hair. John affirms that it was Mary, the sister of Lazarus, while Luke describes a sinful woman
from the city, a prostitute.

The only way John and Luke can both be correct is
if the two disciples are describing entirely different
anointings—one early in Christ's ministry and one
near the end. Since Luke's Gospel was written at least
ten or twenty years before John's, it is highly proba-
ble that John was familiar with Luke's story. Since
the two anointings were so similar, it seems that John
was concerned that the "sinful woman" in Luke's
story might be confused with Mary the sister of
Lazarus. To make sure no such confusion would
exist, John emphasizes his point by twice identifying
Mary as the woman who anointed Jesus in Bethany
six days before the Passover. (Once in John 11:2 and
again in 12:3). Tradition holds that the woman in
Luke's story was Mary Magdalene.

The accounts by Matthew and Mark are almost
identical to one another in every detail, but don't
agree with either Luke or John. Their account is for
another time (two days before the Passover) and in

another house in Bethany (that of Simon the Leper). Matthew and Mark are clearly describing the same incident, but a different one than either of those told by Luke and John.

Taking all of these accounts to be true, we have three instances where Jesus was anointed by a woman with nard and myrrh. Thus, we have three women, in three places, at three times, administering three anointings of Jesus. Two times he was anointed on his feet and once on his head.

That should clarify everything, leaving no contradictions and no discrepancies unreconciled. The mystery of the anointing woman has been solved.

Frankincense and Myrrh

The story of the three wise men coming to see baby Jesus with gifts of frankincense and myrrh causes us to automatically think of one of these two oils when we hear of the other. Earlier in this chapter we mentioned some modern perfumes and colognes containing myrrh. There are also modern fragrances containing frankincense. A perfume actually called "Frankincense and Myrrh," is sold by Czech & Speake in London.

Other commercial fragrances containing frankincense include these feminine perfumes: Replique® (Colonia), Sculptura® (Jovan), Mel® (Frances Denney), Volcan d'Amour® (Diane von Furstenburg), Intreague® (Carven), Cinnabar® (Estee lauder), Youth Dew® (Estee Lauder), and Soir de Paris® (Bourjois) which also contains vetiver and onycha—another Biblical oil.

Contemporary Male fragrances containing frankincense are: Aqua Brava® (Puig), Giorgio® (Giorgio), Jules® (Dior), L'Homme® (Roger & Gallet) and everyone's favorite—Old Spice® (Shulton) which was introduced in 1937 and has been a top-selling mass market fragrance ever since.

Desert Heat and Hippopotamus Fat

Myrrh is like a servant to all the other oils. It is a fixative that increases the longevity of the aroma any fragrance with which it is combined without dominating or overpowering that fragrance. Myrrh is one of those synergistic oils that enhances the qualities of any oil with which it is mixed. But myrrh is a wonderfully healing oil in its own right, and one of the most versatile. It is antiseptic, supports the immune system, enhances the body's natural defenses, helps you relax, helps manage stress and frustration, soothes the skin, is oxygenating to body tissues, is mood elevating, creates a sense of well-being, and promotes overall health, vitality, and longevity.

The Egyptians used myrrh for everything from birth to death and found it to be an effective protection from the desert heat, as well as an insect repellent. Egypt does not receive rain in the region of the lower delta, but the Nile River distributaries create vast wetlands that were breeding grounds for all forms of mosquitoes and other biting insects. Some of these bites could make you sick. Sometimes the sicknesses would end in death. The Egyptians needed ways to protect themselves, not only from the discomfort of the bites and stings, but also from the illnesses they could spread.

Perhaps you have seen pictures of ancient Egyptians with cones on their heads. You may have mistaken these as knots of hair, but they are not. They were lumps of fat from ox, duck, goose, or hippopotamus saturated with myrrh. Sometimes, for variety, they also used oils of marjoram, sweet flag, or lotus. The idea was to place the unguent cone on the top of their heads in the morning and then as the heat rose during the day the fat would melt slowly, running down their half-naked bodies, keeping their skin moist and repelling insects. Sounds pretty yucky to us today, but you have to remember that they had no showers and no screened-in porches. They had to do something, and so they used essential oils like myrrh.

The Many Virtues of Myrrh

According to the *Essential Oils Desk Reference* (EODR), "The Arabian people used myrrh for many skin conditions, such as chapped and cracked skin and wrinkles. It has one of the highest levels of sesquiterpenes (62%), a class of compounds that has direct effects on the hypothalamus, pituitary, and amygdala, the seat of our emotions."

The EODR lists the following indications for myrrh: Bronchitis, diarrhea, dysentery, thrush, ulcers, viral hepatitis, and stretch marks.

Great quantities of myrrh were used by the Romans in their unguents, perfumes, and medicines. Myrrh was also occasionally used in Roman cooking as a spice to encourage appetite. Because of its bitter taste, myrrh can stimulate bile production which pre-pares the digestive tract for processing rich foods—of which the Romans (and Greeks) were very fond.

The oleo-resin of the myrrh tree was also chewed as a gum by the Hebrews and other ancient peoples of the *Bible*. In this way, it helped to prevent infectious diseases of the mouth, teeth, and gums. Even today, myrrh is widely used in oral hygiene products.

Gift of the Wise Men

When Joseph and Mary received the gift of myrrh from the kings of the orient (Matthew 2:11), the wise men did not have to explain the use of the oil to Mary. She knew that the myrrh was antiseptic and should be placed on the navel of the newborn child so that there would be no infection with the sloughing of the umbilical cord. Mary also knew it would come in handy later on in protecting her child from things like coughs, sore throats, thrush, ringworm, and gum infections. She knew myrrh would be a good thing to have to soothe and heal the little cuts and bruises that all little boys experience in their growing up. She knew these things because all of the women of her time knew about these things.

The wise men didn't have to explain to Mary that myrrh could heal scar tissue and remove the stretch marks of pregnancy, either. Mary would have known exactly what to do, to rub her abdomen with the oil until the stretch marks disappeared. All of the women of her time would have known about that, too.

Mary would also have known that the scent of myrrh promotes spiritual awareness and is emotionally uplifting. When rubbed on her body as a breast-feeding mother, it would communicate a sense of security and well-being to both her and her child.

The *Bible* doesn't mention these things because they were common knowledge in that time and their inclusion in the nativity story was not necessary to convey the spiritual purpose of the narrative that Matthew had in mind.

And with this we complete our chapter on the humble and useful oil of myrrh. She not only plays the lead role in the drama of the healing oils of the *Bible*, but she is also the supporting actress and backstage manager—always there to make things happen the way they should, but seldom getting the credit.

Chapter Eleven
Olive: The Other Healing Oil of the Bible

No book on the healing oils of the *Bible* would be complete without a chapter on olive oil. While the word "oil" appears 191 times in the *Bible*, only seven of these are explicit references to olive oil, but in 147 of the 191 references to oil, olive oil can be inferred as the species the writer had in mind. (See Appendix D.)

For the most part, healing oils are essential oils. This is because in order to administer therapy to the body at a cellular level the molecules of an oil must be tiny enough to penetrate into minute spaces. All of the molecules of essential oils are small enough to penetrate human skin, enter the blood stream through the alveolar cells of the lungs, and pass through the blood-brain barrier as well. All of the molecules of essential oils are also tiny enough to act as chemical messengers, unlocking the receptor sites of cells, and communicating with cellular intelligence at the level of the DNA. Molecules of such sizes, all less than 500 amu, are also aromatic and volatile. That is, they evaporate easily, making themselves available to be inhaled and to share their aromas.

Common vegetable oils cannot do this. They are non-aromatic and non-volatile, having little or no fragrance. Their long chain molecules are too large to even penetrate skin to any great depth. As for passing through the microscopic portals that lead into intracellular space, fatty oils cannot do this at all. Most fatty oils have no therapeutic value beyond the surface treatment of chapped, dry, or wounded skin.

Of course, many fatty oils administer therapy by nutrition when eaten, helping to correct many conditions such as cardiovascular disease, etc. While this chapter is going to focus on olive oil, which has some of the healing properties of an essential oil, it is worth noting that consuming walnut and flax seed oils, which were also used in Biblical times, can also have significant healing benefits. (See Appendix D.)

Basically, olive is a fatty oil, an oil for eating, cooking, and burning in lamps, as well as a base oil for anointing. There were other oils pressed from seed in Biblical times—almond, walnut, pistachio, sesame, and flax (or linseed) oils. But none were as popular or as important as olive because olive is different.

First, Beaten, Fine, Virgin, and Extra Virgin

Olive oil comes in two basic grades. The first of them actually contains both fatty and essential oils, making it unique among oils.

When olive oil was extracted in Biblical times, the whole fruit was crushed by a stone wheel (as at Gethsemane) or mashed by treading under foot (as in Micah 6:15). The broken olives were placed in special baskets where the oil was allowed to drain into vats or basins by the force of gravity. This could take a few hours or a day or two. In the *Bible*, the resulting product was called "first oil," "beaten oil," or "fine oil." (Numbers 28:5)

In today's language we call this "virgin oil." The oil that drains in the first hour or so is called "extra virgin," while that which drains later is simply called "virgin." Because the whole fruit is crushed with the hard seed, the result is a mixture of the fatty oil of the seed kernel and the aromatic essential oil of the fruit. Thus, the first oil of the olive is both fatty and essential. Beaten, or virgin, olive oil has a definite and distinct fragrance and flavor due to its aromatic constituents. It also has certain healing properties carried by the essential oils of the olive fruit.

Virgin oils are the most expensive and the most prized by chefs. They are like fine wines where each olive grove and each year's crop produces subtly different nuances of flavor savored by the gourmet. Top grade "first, fine, or beaten" olive oil was also the choice of the Levite priests for offerings, anointing bases, and tithes. (Exodus 27:20; 29:40; Leviticus 24:2; Numbers 28:5)

Second, Pressed, Pure, Refined, Light, and Mild

After the first oil is extracted by simple draining, the crushed olives are then put on a hard surface where heavy stones are stacked upon them to crush them more and press out all of the remaining oil. Systems of levers in stone vats were also used in ancient times, thus gaining a mechanical advantage to press the olives and their seeds. After the last available drops of oil have been squeezed out, along with the juices of the olive pulp, the sediment and water are allowed to settle. The oil is then carefully skimmed off the top. The resulting oil is referred to as the "second," or "pressed," oil of Biblical times.

While draining the olives for first grade oil is a cold process, crushing them under high pressure for second grade oil generates some heat. Since, by this time the aromatic components have either drained into the first oil or have evaporated into the air, pressed olive oil is almost 100% fatty. In today's terminology this is called "pure olive oil." Pure olive oil is derived purely from the hard seed and not the fruit. It has no fragrance and no taste and no therapeutic value.

Second oil was less expensive in Biblical times (as it still is today) and was used by the poorer masses for household lighting and food. By comparison, the temples and tabernacles would accept only virgin or fine oil for their lamps and sacrifices and for the food offerings eaten by the Levite priests and their families. (See Priest's Due in Appendix D.)

There are other grades of olive oils. There is a refined grade that is second oil heated to remove every trace of any aromatic left in order to produce a truly neutral or flavorless oil. This grade is called "refined olive oil."

There are also "light" and "mild" grades. These are pressed grade oils with some virgin oil added to lend a light or mild aroma and flavor. These grades of oil are generally less expensive than virgin oil and more expensive than pure pressed oil.

In order to retain the aromatic, or essential, components of olive oil, it must not be heated as in frying. It is best eaten cold, as a salad oil, or dipped with bread (as in Biblical times) as a substitute for butter like on pop corn. It can also be added to soups and dishes while warm after they have been cooked.

Staple of the Holy Land

The olive as a fruit and the oil it produced were mainstays of the Hebrew diet from Genesis through the *New Testament*. Olives were a staple for the early Christians as well. Even today the olive is a principal source of food and cooking oil to most of the countries that border the Mediterranean from the Holy Land to the Straits of Gibraltar. It's attractive wood was also prized for carvings and temple doors. (I Kings 6:23, 31-33)

Olive trees have been cultivated for thousands of years from ancient Egypt to the present. They were ubiquitous to the Biblical landscape. 1,250 years before Christ, Moses described the promised land in Deuteronomy 8:8 as "A land of olive trees and honey."

Olive trees live exceedingly long. Even when cut to the ground they usually sprout back to form new trees from old roots. Although the Romans destroyed the groves that covered the Mount of Olives in August of 70 A.D., there are olive trees living there today thought to have risen from the roots of those beneath which Jesus prayed and gathered his disciples 2,000 years ago. (Matthew 26:36; Mark 14:26; John 8:1)

It is a spiritual and symbolic irony that after the Romans tried to silence Christ by crucifixion, he arose from the grave and continues to care and nurture us to the present day. At the same time, some of the very trees beneath which he was arrested have resurrected with new life that also continues to serve and shelter us today—2,000 years after the Romans tried to destroy them.

While Christians make pilgrimages to the Mount of Olives because of its relationship to Jesus, its Biblical significance dates well before the days of Solomon. King David prayed and wept there 1,000 years before Christ, no doubt, beneath some of the same olive trees that sheltered Jesus. (II Samuel 15:30)

The Olive Tree as Legend

Olive trees (olea europea) are attractive evergreens with a distinctive gnarled trunk. Their lancelet leaves are bluish green on one side and silvery white on the other. They seem to be one of God's special creations for the benefit of mankind. It is probably significant that the very first evidence of new life following the Great Flood was an olive branch. (Genesis 8:11) There is even a Rabbinic tradition claiming that the dove obtained the branch brought to Noah from the Mount of Olives.

To the Israelites the olive tree and its gifts assumed an almost mythical character. In Psalms 128:3 it was a symbol of fertility. In Jeremiah 11:16 and Hosea 14:6 it represented fairness and beauty. To Noah and his family it represented peace and bountifulness. (Genesis 8:11). And, of course, the olive tree became inextricably associated with Jesus by his many visits to Olivet. The Garden of Gethsemane, which was located on the Mount, was a place where olives and grapes were grown and processed. In fact, the literal meaning of Gethsemane in Hebrew is "wine and oil press." (Matthew 26:36; Mark 14:26, 32; Luke 22:39-46; John 8:1)

Health Benefits of Olive Oil

Everyone agrees, from Hebrews to Hippocrates, olive oil is #1. According to Dr. Andrew Weil (MD), author of several books on health and longevity, "Olive oil is the best and safest of all oils," and he adds, "It tastes good, too." The virgin or beaten oil of the *Bible* is predominantly monounsaturated fats containing a small percent of essential oils of the fruit. Most other vegetable oils are predominantly polyunsaturated and contain no essential oils. Numerous studies have shown that daily intake of olive oil significantly reduces the incidence of heart disease of all kinds, including death by heart attack. Olive oil has been shown to thin the blood, lower blood pressure, and regulate cholesterol by reducing the bad kind (LDL) while maintaining the good kind (HDL). It has been observed for centuries that the cultures around the Mediterranean Sea, including the residents of the Holy Land, have significantly lower rates of heart attack, as well as lower rates of many other degenerative and disabling diseases. Experts agree that olive oil is the common factor in all of these cultures.

According to Dr. Weil, the high level of health and longevity of people in the Mediterranean region may have to do with the fact that they "eat plenty of fruits and vegetables, whole grain breads, substantial quantities of fish, and only moderate amounts of animal foods, but," he continues, "when all of these factors are analyzed, olive oil has the highest correlation with better health than any other factor."

"If the only change you make in your diet is to replace butter and margarine with olive oil," Weil concludes, "you will have made a tremendous step toward better health and healing."

According to Jean Carper, author of *The Food Pharmacy*, "One tablespoon of olive oil has the power to wipe out the cholesterol raising effects of two eggs." Olive oil is known to cleanse and assist liver function, regulate bile production, and reduce the incidence of gall stones. Olive oil also helps to restore normal digestion and even to help in the healing of certain types of ulcers. Daily intake of olive oil has also been observed to have anti-inflammatory benefits for arthritis pain, lubricating the joints and reducing swelling. And finally, mainly because of its aromatic oil content, olive oil is an effective antioxidant that has been shown to reduce cancer rates and increase longevity.

Whether the people of Biblical times knew all of this or not, we don't know. We do know that olive oil was a staple of their daily diets. They dipped their bread in it (instead of using butter), mixed it with their foods, and cooked with it. By burning it in their lamps, they also diffused a certain amount of essential olive oil vapors in their homes and tabernacles, which may have also had aromatherapeutic benefits.

Eating Olive Oil for Wellness and Longevity

If you are to use olive oil for its health benefits, you need to follow the example of the Levite priests and insist on virgin or extra virgin oil, the grade with the full-bodied flavor and aroma of the essential oils of olive. When offerings and tithes were brought to the temple, the Levites kept back the majority of the oils and products for consumption by themselves and their families. This is the only income or support the priests were allowed to receive. In return for their spiritual service, the officials of the Jewish temples, tabernacles, and synagogues were to receive only the most healthful grades of olive oils, as well as the best of all offerings, including fruits, grains, vegetables, and meat. (Leviticus 2:3, 10; Deuteronomy 18:3-8; Nehemiah 13:5)

A properly derived virgin oil is cold pressed, which preserves its aromatic content. When using olive oil for its dietary benefits, heating the oil, as in frying, destroys the essential content and can alter the molecular structure of the remaining fatty oils such that its healthful properties are lost. If you wish to have olive oil in a hot dish or soup, add it after the cooking is completed.

From Hebrews to Hippocrates

Twenty-five hundred years ago, Hippocrates said, "Let your food be your medicine and your medicine be your food." Olive oil is a perfect example of such a food. Taken internally as a food it is not only good preventative medicine, it is also healing in many ways, as mentioned earlier in this chapter. Olive oil has also been used externally as a healing ointment for thousands of years by Greeks, Romans, Egyptians, Christians, and Jews. While usually combined with essential oils, it was routinely applied to cuts, sores, bleeding wounds, bruises, and injuries of all kinds, often with a little wine as an antiseptic.

In Isaiah 1:6 we read of "oil" or "ointment" being applied to wounds, bruises, and sores. In this instance the Hebrew word used is "shemen" which often implies a combination of olive oil containing essential oils from spices, including cinnamon or cassia, both of which are highly antiseptic.

Luke, the physician, recounts Jesus' parable of the Good Samaritan who finds a man beaten by thieves and binds up his wounds, "pouring in oil and wine." (Luke 10:34) Here, the Greek word "elion" implies an olive oil base containing aromatic oils as was the custom of the time. It would not be uncommon, in those days, for travelers, such as the Good Samaritan, to carry a quantity of wine containing myrrh along with a flask of scented olive oil wherever they went.

In addition to the health and healing properties possessed by olive oil in its own right, it was the most commonly used Biblical base for applying essential oils. The foregoing discussion shows that olive oil as a base is much more than a passive carrier. Along with the healing aromatics with which it may be blended, it is, in fact, also an active participant in the healing process. Thus we call it, "The Other Healing Oil of the *Bible*."

NOTE: Appendix D is a catalogue of *Bible* references to Olive Oil.

Chapter 12
Extracting Essences
In Biblical Times

Essential oils are the water immiscible, lipid soluble portion of the plant juices that give it fragrance, flavor, character, and life. Essential oils are found in leaves, stems, roots, branches, bark, flowers, fruits, and oleo-gum-resins. You may recall from Chapter Two that by strict technical definitions the "gum" of the plant fluid is water soluble, the "resin" is alcohol soluble, and the "oleo" part is the oil which is soluble in any oil, fat, or lipid. There is a brief discussion at the beginning of Chapter Two on extracting the gum with water, the resin with alcohol (wine), and the oleo by various means. In this chapter we shall focus mainly on the extraction and concentration of the oil.

Fresh Plants as Medicines

A fresh plant contains every constituent of the oleo-gum-resin, as well as natural chemicals bonded to the tissues of the plant. Eating a live plant would deliver almost all that it has to offer to your system, including its fiber. Drinking the juice of a fresh plant would provide you with almost all of the oleo-gum-resin. But in the fresh juice of a plant, the oils would be in a diluted form since most plants contain less than 2% oil and some less than 1%.

The distillation of an oil from a plant normally concentrates the oils from their original state by 50 to 100 times. For some plants, like melissa or the petals of roses, the concentration from nature is even greater, and can be as much as 5,000 times. This is why oils such as these are so expensive. This is also why even one breath of the concentrated fragrance or one drop of the oil can be so effective as an agent of healing.

Not all plants contain useful percentages of oil and yet they may have healing properties. Some highly effective medicinal plants (such as mushrooms) contain no oil at all. Fresh and whole plants have therapeutic benefits not available from oils or dried herbs. Therefore, the art and science of using plants as medicines for health and healing includes gathering and using fresh materials.

Dried Herbs as Medicines

A dried herb contains the heavier, non-volatile oils (triterpenes and tetraterpenes) and the precipitated residues of evaporated fluids, but will be missing 95% of the aromatic oils. The heavy, non-volatile lipid soluble constituents (which are not found in essential oils) are concentrated in the dried herb.

Dried herbs can be stored for long periods of time without losing their potency because they are in a state of restful sleep. They can be awakened and their healing constituents effectively absorbed into our systems by brewing teas and by other means. The teas may be drunk, applied as rinses to the skin, or used to create hot poultices for transdermal or inhalation applications.

Dried herbs have unique healing properties not found in fresh plants or essential oils. Therefore, the art and science of using plants as medicines for health and healing also includes gathering herbs, drying them, and brewing teas for various purposes.

Essential Oils as Medicines

Essential oils are concentrates of the oleo, or lipid soluble, aromatic portion of a plant's life fluids. When the oils are extracted by steam distillation, the larger oil molecules remain behind with the plant fiber because they are too large to pass through the vapor stage of the distillation process.

The potent concentrations of essential oils combined with their unique capabilities to pass through all the tissues of the body and interact positively with cellular intelligence, plus their ability to make direct contact with our emotions and awaken past memories, sets them apart from all other natural medicines.

Therefore, the art and science of using plants as medicines for health and healing, as directed by God in Ezekiel 47:12, must include the extracting and application of essential oils.

Thus we see that the plant kingdom offers countless varieties of medicines created by God—sufficient to address every ailment known to humankind. Instead of spending billions on secular profit-motivated research to create new synthetic drugs, antibiotics, vaccines, and surgical procedures, our research should be toward discovering, studying, and applying the vast array of medicines that God has already perfected in forms already available to us.

When prayer becomes an integral part of the scientific method and we learn to include God as a partner in our research, he will guide us to the solutions for every condition. These are solutions he has already prepared, that merely await our recognition and discovery. Once society realizes that God is the sole source of all healing, his remedies will become evident and available and the need for pharmaceuticals and allopathic medicine will all but vanish.

Steam Distillation

Essential oils were extracted or otherwise made available for human use in a variety of ways. With yields of 1-2%, a hundred pounds of plant material would yield 1-2 pounds of oil. For exotic oils like rose, whose oil content is only .02-.04%, it takes 3,000-5,000 pounds of petals to produce one pound of oil.

Among the ancient Hebrews, the art of creating anointing oils, incense, perfumes, and medicinal ointments was the responsibility of the Jewish priesthood. The priests may have also engaged in extracting oils from plants but probably obtained most of their ingredients from secular producers and trading merchants who engaged in the international commercial trade of those times. Keeping a supply of the incense and anointing oils needed for daily use in the temple was up to the priests. They are referred to as "apothecaries" and "perfumers" in the *Bible*. (Exodus 30:25, 35; 37:29; II Chronicles 16:14; Nehemiah 3:8; Ecclesiastes 10:1)

In steam distillation, plant parts (leaves, flowers, stems, roots, resins, etc.) were packed into a vessel through which steam was passed at atmospheric pressure for several hours. The steam vapors absorbed the aromatic molecules in the plant and passed them through a tube into a condensation vat where the oils would separate from the water, usually floating to the top, where they were skimmed off. This process produced not only a pure essential oil, but a volume of water, called a hydrosol or floral water, containing the water soluble portions of the plant juices along with traces of emulsified oil.

Hydrosols are not mentioned in the *Bible*, but because they are healthful and contain healing properties they were probably used.

Steam distillation is a process known to have been used by Babylonians, Chinese, East Indians, Egyptians, and Sumerians at least as far back as 3500 B.C. One of the earliest oils extracted by the Egyptians and Sumerians was cedarwood. The distilled essences of frankincense and myrrh have also been widely used since the earliest times of antiquity.

As the general knowledge and understanding of the world declined into the Dark Ages from 1000 B.C. through the time of Christ, the technology of distillation gradually became lost. By the fall of Rome in 500 A.D., it was lost entirely. Four or five centuries later it was rediscovered by Avicenna, an Arabian physician. One of the first oils produced from his still was rose, which soon gave rise to an Arabian perfume trade for that highly esteemed fragrance, a trade that has flourished for a thousand years ever since. Avicenna also found the hydrosol from distilled rose oil of great therapeutic benefit and wrote a book on it.

Steam distillation in Biblical times were in stills made of stone and pottery, which were ideal materials inasmuch as rock and ceramic are chemically inert in response to the oils. Some modern stills are made of metals that contaminate the oils. However, certain types of stainless steel are non-reactive and can be used to build stills that produce oils with the same therapeutic purity as was produced by the Biblical apothecaries. Steam distillation was the best way to produce a pure essential oil in ancient times, and it still is today.

Maceration

A defining property of essential oil is its solubility in other oils. Maceration was an ancient method of extracting essential oils by immersing plant material in a heavier oil or fat, thus dissolving the lipid soluble portion of the plant fluid. One of the main oils used by the Egyptians for this purpose was castor bean oil, but they also used goose, ox, crocodile and even hippopotamus fat. Various vegetable oils were also used in Biblical times such as almond, walnut, flax seed or pistachio. The Hebrews also used goat fat and, of course, olive oil. The kings and queens of the *Old Testament* received "spiced olive oil" in massages.

A common technique was to pack a vessel with the herb (crushed leaves, flowers, stems, seeds, etc.) and then pour in the oil to the top, usually warmed or heated. After several days, or even weeks, the oily mash was then strained or squeezed through linen and a perfumed oil was the result—a blend of both fatty and essential oils. Sometimes the scented oil would again be packed with fresh herbal material. This process could be repeated until the desired concentration was obtained. The final product would again be strained through several linens to remove all the plant sediment and debris. The result was a fine perfume, unguent, or ointment.

Maceration does not result in a pure essential oil as does steam distillation. But for many applications (such as massage, anointing, or medicine) pure essential oils are blended with carrier oils anyhow. Maceration produces a blended and diluted product ready to use.

The essences of rose, narcissus, and jasmine were often extracted by Biblical perfumers by maceration. While the oil of rose petals can be successfully extracted by distillation, the light constituents of jasmine are so fragile and delicate that any heat would chemically alter and destroy the scent. Hence, a cold process like maceration was the only way to extract it in ancient times. Today, oils such as jasmine are often extracted by chemical solvents.

Expressed Oils

Another way oils can be extracted from plant material is by expression. When essential oils are expressed (squeezed) from plant material under pressure, the larger molecules (triterpenes and tetraterpenes) remain in the resulting oil, molecules too large to pass through a distillation process.

In aromatherapy today, only the oils from the rinds of citrus fruits are expressed. This includes orange, grapefruit, lemon, lime, tangerine, bergamot, and mandarin. Citrus oils are also distilled from bitter orange flowers (neroli) and orange tree leaves and twigs (petitgrain).

While second grade olive oil and other fatty oils of the *Bible* were obtained by expression (see Chapter 11), expressed essential oils were unknown in Biblical times. Citrus fruits and trees, which originated in the Orient, were also unknown to the West and Middle East until more than 1,000 years after Christ. The process of expressing (or pressing) oils was reserved for the fatty oils of Biblical times. Most essential oils do not express well because they are too light and evaporate too readily. Citrus oils can be expressed only because they contain heavy molecules.

Enfleurage

While expression, as such, was not a common means of accessing essential oils in Biblical times, sometimes a combination of maceration and pressing was used. The process is called enfleurage and is one of the most ancient of methods.

Flower petals, or other plant materials, were placed in a trough containing a base oil (like olive) through which a heavy stone was rolled, crushing the plant tissues and releasing their oils to be dissolved in the carrier base.

This process could yield a greater percent of essential oil in less time than the simpler method of soaking in pots for days at a time. However, some of the fragrance was lost by evaporation due to exposure to the air in the pressing-crushing operation.This process was used extensively in producing rose oils.

Infusion

Infusion is a variation of maceration where aromatic plant materials or spices are packed in oil and then heated to get more rapid extraction and, perhaps, more of the essential oil out into the carrier. Heating could be by fire or by sunlight on a rooftop. Delicate aromas, such as jasmine, would not withstand such heating, however,

Infusion was particularly used when the maceration base oil was a fat that was solid at room temperatures. In this way, the cooled down product was a solid salve or unguent.

Since the term "spices" in Biblical terminology could refer to solid or ground plant materials as well as to oils distilled from aromatic plants, it is not clear in Exodus 30:23-25 whether the holy anointing oil described there was a mixture of distilled oils mixed with olive, or whether the cassia, calamus, cinnamon, and myrrh were in plant or resinous forms to be macerated by the olive oil. Regardless of the form, whether solid or liquid, the spiciness of a spice is in the oil it contains. Either way, the result was a blend of essential oils in a carrier base.

Fumigation

Another way to release essential oils for human absorption is by vaporizing or burning and inhaling the fumes or smoke. By today's standards, we would consider this practice wasteful. It is not a very efficient way to make oils available to our bodies. The heat destroys some of the medicinal value.

Cold diffusion is much better, but was a technology unavailable in Biblical times. Electrically powered nebulizing diffusers are the most efficient means of filing the air with essential oil molecules but such devices have only become available in very recent times.

Nevertheless, inhaling the fumes of burning aromatic plants, or the vapors of incense, does bring molecules of essential oils into our systems quite effectively. Of course, the portions of the plant that actually burn (oxidize) have been chemically changed from their natural state. However, the smoke contains substantial quantities of vaporized oil that have not been chemically altered. Technically, this means of delivering essential oils to our systems is called "fumigation."

In fact, the word "perfume" comes from the Latin "per fumum" which means "through smoke." The word "fume" is also derived from the same root and and originally referred to the aromatic vapors of smoldering oil or incense from a censer.

How Effective is Fumigation?

The effectiveness of this means of delivery of natural plant products is well known to those who smoke tobacco, marijuana, or opium. Smoking is, in fact, a form of aromatherapy. Those who engage in it derive benefits they value or they would not choose to do it. These benefits are usually on an emotional level or in the realm of pleasure, but they also include stimulation of adrenaline, reduction of anxiety, pain relief, alleviation of nervousness, and curbing of appetite, which are all forms of therapy.

Of course, there are well known undesirable side effects to smoking, not the least of which are emphysema, pleurisy, breast cancer, birth defects, and lung cancer. Nevertheless, smoking is a form of absorbing essential oils through the lungs and nasal passages, which is the defining feature of aromatherapy. It is not a version we recommend, however, nor was it widely used in the Biblical world. Opium pipe smoking was practiced in China for thousands of years, a practice that found its way to a limited extent into ancient Persia and Arabia. But as for the peoples of the *Bible*, they didn't smoke.

It is interesting to note that the world's largest consumer of clove isn't the flavoring or cooking spice industry, but the tobacco industry. Oil of clove, though not mentioned in the *Bible*, has been used in and around the Holy Land for thousands of years. (See Appendix C.) Clove is one of the most effective of natural anesthetics. Cigarette manufacturers add many ingredients to their products to improve taste. Because of its ability to numb the tongue, clove is added to many cigarettes to reduce the bite and take away the sting, thus producing a smoother taste. Paradoxically, a little clove oil on the tongue can help break a smoking habit.

Aaron Stops a Plague

In Biblical times, the most common form of fumigation was the burning or vaporizing of incense, which was required twenty-four hours a day in the temples and tabernacles. (Exodus 30:8) The holy incense of Exodus 30:34-36 was one of many formulas burned by the ancient Hebrews. Other types of incense were burned in their homes and businesses.

In addition to its use in temple worship, the holy

incense of the Hebrews was also highly effective as a preventative against disease. In Numbers 16:46-50, we read the following:

> "Moses said to Aaron, "Take your censer, put fire on it from the altar, and lay incense on it, and carry it quickly to the congregation and make atonement for them. For wrath has gone out from the Lord; the plague has begun.' So Aaron took it as Moses had ordered, and ran into the middle of the assembly, where the plague had already begun among the people. He put on the incense, and made atonement for the people. He stood between the dead and the living; and the plague was stopped. Those who died by the plague were fourteen thousand seven hundred, besides those who died in the affair of Korah. When the plague was stopped, Aaron returned to Moses at the entrance of the tent of meeting." (Numbers 16:46-50)

The incense referred to in this passage is "quetoreth," which was the holy incense of Exodus 30:34-37 containing frankincense, galbanum, onycha, and myrrh. Censers (also called thuribles) were vented metal or ceramic containers in which hot coals were placed that were carried and swung from a chain. (See silver vessel on front cover and caption on p. vi.) They came in various ornate shapes, including figures of birds and animals. Aromatic oils, spices, or incense were dropped onto the coals or placed on a shelf over the coals to create a fragrant smoke. Censers are mentioned 20 times in the *Bible*. (Appendix A, Table 4-A.)

When Aaron "ran into the middle of the assembly," this was not something that took place in a few minutes or hours. The Israelites numbers in the hundreds of thousands. It probably took days, even weeks, for Aaron and his sons to distribute the therapeutic fumes to every tent, dwelling, and campsite of the congregation. However long it must have taken, it was effective. The plague was stopped, along with the death and the dying. Today, we understand from a scientific point of view how fumigating with essential oils such as these could kill a virus or stop a bacteria.

Smudging

Another fumigation technique applied for healing purposes in ancient times was smudging. The aromatic oil, gum, or dried herb is placed on a hot coal or other heat source, and the smoke or fumes are blown, or fanned, and aimed at specific places on the body such as the feet, face, head, locations along the spine, or specific diseased areas. Warm vapors of essential oil can actually be directly absorbed through the skin by this technique. When blowing near the face, the patient is instructed to inhale deeply as much as possible.

Native Americans have used this technique for thousands of years and still use it today. In Biblical times, the Greeks, Romans and Egyptians smudged with oils of cedarwood, juniper, myrrh and others as deemed appropriate to the needs of the receiver. It is possible and likely that the Hebrew physicians also used smudging as well, although this technique is not identified in the *Old* or *New Testament*s.

The midwives of Biblical times used a variation of smudging during childbirth. Hot coals were placed under the beds or birthing stools of laboring women. Myrrh and other oils were poured on to create a cloud of perfumed smoke around the mother. This was supposed to assist in keeping her calm and focused on the task at hand and to ease the stress of labor.

Tread, Crush, and Bruise

When we want to test the fragrance of an herb or plant, we instinctively pluck a leaf or break off a part of the stalk, crush it between our thumbs and fingers and hold it to our noses. By this simple process the oils of the plant are released into the atmosphere where they reach our sense of smell. Application of this idea was other way aromatic oils were applied in Biblical times. The Hebrews would scatter fresh leaves, twigs, or flowers on the floor. Then, by their mere walking, fragrant oils would be released into the air. This form of accessing plant oils, although it involved crushing, was not the same as expression or pressing out essential oils with a fatty oil to be collected in liquid form. This means of diffusing natural oils put them directly into the air as vapors to be immediately inhaled.

The Jewish places of worship used the leaves and stems of fresh mint, marjoram, and other herbs in this way. They would sprinkle the chopped plant parts on the hard stone floors so that when people walked on them, they would be crushed and bruised, releasing their fragrances and freshening the air.

Cleansing the atmosphere was especially important in the temples where they sacrificed animals on a daily basis. The stench of burning flesh, hair, and feathers must have been difficult to bear. A bit of mint in the air would have been a welcome relief—particularly for the Levites who would have smelled the worst of it. The essence of mint and other oils in the air would also have been a disinfectant, protecting those who visited the temple from the spread of disease.

Another Biblical example of bruising leaves to release fragrances is found in the story of the passover:

> "And you shall take a bunch of hyssop, and dip it in the blood that is in the basin, and strike the lintel and the two side posts. . ." (Exodus 12:22)

The "striking" of the lintel and the posts of the doorways would have bruised the aromatic leaves of the hyssop, thus releasing the fragrance of its oil. The fragrance of hyssop was thought, by the ancient Israelites, to repel evil spirits. On that particular eve, it was the angel of death they sought to dissuade from entering their dwellings.

So we see that, in *Bible* times, essential oils were unlocked and released from the plants that contained them in at least seven general ways:

1. By Distillation
2. By Maceration
3. By Enfleurage
4. By Infusion
5. By Burning
6. By Vaporization
7. By Crushing/Bruising

Modern Methods

While distillation is the most common means of obtaining essential oils today, in modern times, new methods of essential oil extraction have been developed that were unknown and unavailable in ancient times. The perfume and flavoring industries, who produce more than 90% of the essential oils used today, like to use high temperature, high pressure distillation techniques because they are more economical. However, this process destroys the therapeutic properties of the oil and makes it unfit for healing purposes. (See Chapter 13.)

Another modern innovation is the use of chemical solvents to extract the oils, including the use of solvents after distillation, to squeeze every last droplet of oil from the plant. These include hexane and other petrochemicals that are toxic. Traces of these chemicals unavoidably remain in the resultant essential oil extracts. Such oils are not suitable for healing purposes, and, except for trace amounts in foods, shampoos, soaps, or cosmetics, they are toxic and harmful to humans. Here, again, the motive is economics and not therapeutic quality. Using solvents reduces costs and increases profits, but it cannot produce a healing oil. Such processes were never used in Biblical times because the chemical industry did not yet exist.

Another modern method of extraction is called "carbon dioxide distillation." This is an expensive process performed at cold temperatures, approximately 40°--50° below zero Fahrenheit (minus 40°-45° Celsius). These are the temperatures where carbon dioxide gas become the solid known as "dry ice." This method of extraction results in an extremely pure essential oil containing no adulterants and retaining a larger bouquet of lighter constituents than can be retained by steam distillation or by any other means known. Oils obtained by CO_2 extraction are therapeutic in grade. Such oils, with their broader spectrum of aromatic constituents, are expected to become more available in time as the economics of the procedure can be refined and brought to a more affordable level.

In summary, the healing oils of the *Bible* had healing properties because they were organically grown or gathered wild and thus uncontaminated by chemicals of any kind. Furthermore, they were gently extracted to preserve their life force and therapeutic constituents. To obtain oils with the same healing potentials as those of the *Bible*, one must find growers and distillers and honest retailers who follow the Biblical traditions.

Chapter 13
Oils that Heal Versus Oils that Don't

In order for pure essential oils to be of therapeutic grade, they must be derived from organically grown or wildcrafted plants. They must be steam distilled at atmospheric pressures and minimum temperatures in vessels that are non-reactive. And they must be bottled in dark or opaque non-reactive containers with no adulteration, dilution, refinement or tampering with the oils in any way as they come from the still. Exceptions to this include certain oils that are not steam distilled, but are pressed, such as those from the rinds of certain fruits.

In Biblical times, the vessels of distillation were of stone or fired pottery. In modern times the best non-reactive material is stainless steel. Copper is sometimes used (and was available in Biblical times) but it can contaminate the oil with a heavy metal. In Biblical times oils were stored in fired pottery jars or boxes carved from alabaster. In modern times the best non-reactive containers are of dark glass with teflon or non-reactive, air-tight plastic tops. In Biblical times the necessary air-tight seals were achieved by waxes poured over the oils in their containers. These hard wax covers had to be broken to gain access to the liquid oil within.

The reason for the dark glass is a protection from light that causes oils to polymerize, increasing the size of their molecules, and, thus, destroying their capability to penetrate human tissue and bring about healing. Polymerized oils lose their fragrance, their molecules having become too large to evaporate and enter the nose.

The necessity of the air-tight seals on oil containers is two-fold. When exposed to the air, the most volatile components of the oils readily escape. This reduces the medicinal value of the oil inasmuch as the lightest ingredients often contain the greatest capabilities to heal. Oils must also be protected from exposure to the atmosphere to prevent oxidation, which chemically alters the nature of the oil. Oxidized oils lose their therapeutic qualities. Their fragrances are also changed, thus destroying their value as perfumes.

Unless an essential oil has met all of the above criteria for production and storage, it is not of therapeutic grade and is not, therefore, a healing oil.

How Modern Techniques Destroy Oils

When plants are grown commercially with pesticides, herbicides, and chemicals (to save on agricultural costs), or when they are distilled at too high a temperature and pressure (to cut processing time and reduce production costs), or when they are extracted with chemical solvents (to squeeze more product from the plant than it wishes to volunteer on its own), the result is an oil with compromised life force or, perhaps, no life at all.

For such oils, most of the chemical components of the original God-created oil may still be present, which leads pharmaceutically minded scientists to conclude that these oils produced by modern means are "essentially" the same as oils produced by the more expensive and painstaking methods that emulate the ancient traditions.

What they fail to appreciate is that the most important constituents of a healing oil are often only present in trace amounts that cannot be measured by even the best of laboratory equipment, yet their presence, like the traces of enzymes necessary to maintain the functions of our bodies, is crucial to the ability of the oil to function therapeutically.

Furthermore, properly extracted essential oils have the highest known electromagnetic frequencies of any known substances, ranging from 52-320 Megahertz (MHz). Besides their chemical benefits, essential oils also heal by raising our bodily electromagnetic frequencies. (See Chapter Two on "How and Why Oils Can Heal.") Tampering with God's natural oils reduces their frequencies such that they are no longer able to elevate our human frequencies and, thus, are no longer able to heal in that way.

Furthermore, when synthetic compounds are added (to restore some of the fragrance components lost in high-pressure distillation), or when oils are "refined" (i.e. certain constituents are removed to manipulate the oil into a particular formula to fit a perfume standard, to meet a flavor grade, or to make up a deficiency created by improper production techniques), or when oils are diluted (to increase the volume and the profit to the distributor) their therapeutic value is reduced or removed altogether. In fact, such manipulation poisons the oil, lowers its electromagnetic frequency, and kills its life force. Dead oils cannot heal. They may still have a fragrance or flavor to satisfy the perfumers and food makers, but they are not therapeutic grade oils.

Fraud in the Oil Industry

When oils are grown, distilled, and processed by the most economic and expeditious means, as described above, it is not fraud when such oils are sold and used for flavorings and fragrances. In fact, it is because these industries demand the lowest prices and require certain gross chemical standards for their oils that all of these methods of farming and processing have been developed, accepted, and used. The demand for therapeutic grade oils is miniscule by comparison, comprising less than 5% of the market. The short cuts taken by the food and fragrance industries in producing essential oils only become fraud when their products are sold as "therapeutic," when, in fact, they are not. (Also see section on "Commercial Christian Anointing Oils" on pp. 218-220)

Because true healing oils are expensive to produce the temptation to commit fraud is rampant in the industry, which is why you want to purchase oils from producers where you can identify the grower, the distiller and the packager. Anywhere along this production chain, from growing soil to bottled oil, tampering can occur to increase profits. To make matters worse, there are no well regulated labeling laws in the United States as there are in Europe.

What Labels Really Mean

You can find oils in retail stores whose labels say things like "100% pure, organic, and natural." They may even say "therapeutic grade." Most of the time, this would be an outright lie, but a legal one since no government agency has defined the term "therapeutic" and no government agency, as yet, regulates the content of labels on essential oils in a way that would remedy such deceptions.

As for "100%" that quantitative term does not really mean 100%. In some cases 100% can mean as little as 10% of the real stuff while the rest may be a colorless, odorless petrochemical. Yet this is tolerated as okay in the retail trade.

Another misleading term is the word "organic." Educated health-oriented people interpret that to mean "grown naturally without poisons or chemicals." But the definition of "organic," as used by organic chemists, is that organic means "composed of carbon compounds." In other words, any carbon compound is "organic."

By this definition, most pharmaceuticals (and all petrochemicals) are "organic," regardless of their origin. In other words, gasoline is organic. Pure rubbing alcohol is organic. Dioxin, a known carcinogen, is organic. Highly toxic industrial solvents such benzene, hexane, toluene, xylene, and carbon tetrachloride are organic. By this definition, every artificial compound synthesized by an organic chemical laboratory is "organic." So when these adulterants are added to an essential oil, the term "organic" can still legally be used, implying one thing to an organic chemist yet something quite different to an unsuspecting customer.

Some of the dilutants used in essential oils are odorless, colorless petrochemicals (which are cheap). However, such compounds can be harmful to one's health when applied to the skin, taken internally, or inhaled over long periods of time. The common availability of such adulterated oils has caused some aromatherapists, who unsuspectingly and routinely use such products, to conclude that it is not safe to use an essential oil directly (neat) without diluting it down to a 2-5% concentration in a neutral fatty base. If such aromatherapists would seek out a reliable source of truly pure therapeutic grade oils, they would find that applying essential oils neat is perfectly safe (with a few exceptions) and of far greater therapeutic value than using them diluted.

Understanding English

There is also another labeling phrase you will see that can be misleading: "aromatherapy grade." This is actually a term of British origin and is okay and understood in that country.

In Great Britain the practice of aromatherapy is principally the practice of massage with oils. Hence, an "aromatherapy grade" oil is one that is 95-98% massage oil, such a grape seed, jojoba, almond, or some other fatty oil, and only 2-5% essential oil, which can be food or fragrance grade, and still fulfill the English requirements. The phrase is clearly understood in England to mean diluted, but misunderstood in America to mean pure or therapeutic essential oil. It is a matter of differentiating between American English and British English. When understood, an oil labeled as "aromatherapy grade" can be recognized as an adulterated/diluted oil, by definition, and probably unfit for therapeutic use.

British aromatherapists generally never apply essential oils neat to the skin for fear of toxic reactions. In fact, most British users of essential oils are horrified at the thought of applying pure essential oils to the body and disbelieve that Esther of the *Bible* (Esther 2:12) really rubbed pure oil of myrrh over her body for six months in preparation for her marriage to the king. This fear, peculiar to the English and to those who study under them or read their writings, is because most British essential oils are by-products of the food and fragrance industry, which are not therapeutic. Such oils probably are toxic if used neat. Used in minute amounts in foods and perfumes, and diluted for massage, there are usually no serious toxic reactions.

British aromatherapists do not report the healings

that are common where therapeutic grade oils are used neat, as in the U.S., France, and elsewhere.

What is USP or BP Grade Oil?

The labels of some American oils say "Pure USP Grade Oil" while in Great Britain some say "Pure BP Grade." USP means "United States Pharmacopeia." BP means "British Pharmacopeia." In both instances, this is in reference to a set of standards for essential oils set by the food and fragrance industries. These standards are set so that successive batches of oil will be the same, or as nearly identical as can be made possible. In order to get lavender oil, for example, to always have the same proportions of its major constituents the oil producer must refine it or denature it (i.e. remove excessive or unwanted compounds) or add synthetic compounds to bring the proportions "up to standard." In other words, a USP or BP grade oil is, by definition, an altered and adulterated oil and not therapeutic. Such oils are intended for foods and perfumes, not for healing.

When is "Natural" Natural?

Another subterfuge to fool the trusting oil shopper is the word, "natural." Any compound that can be produced synthetically by a laboratory that is also found in nature can be legally labeled and sold as "natural," even though the process by which it was produced was totally unnatural and the raw products from which it was manufactured may have been petroleum, coal, or natural gas.

A comparative chemical analysis of the synthetic and the natural component would be identical for a specific compound, such as methyl salicylate, whether produced in a chemical factory or by a wintergreen plant (*Galtheria procumbens*), or a birch tree

(*Betula alleghaniansis*). But the synthetically produced version will not have the same isomeric mix as
the naturally produced version. In other words, the
same proportions of carbon, hydrogen, and oxygen
will be present in both the manufactured and the natural methyl salicylate, but the assortment of struc-
tural arrangements at a molecular level will be different, thus giving the two seemingly "identical" compounds different properties when applied to the
human body. Since precise determinations of isomeric proportions are difficult and often impossible, the
true composition of a natural ingredient of an oil can
not be duplicated.

Chemistry Isn't Everything

Furthermore, the living element or electromagnetic
frequency present in the natural oils of wintergreen
and birch is absent in the synthetically produced version. Thus, all pertinent factors are not considered by
chemists in synthesizing an oil. Electromagnetic frequency is another factor they cannot duplicate. A
chemical analysis, however meticulous, isn't sufficient
to adequately describe a therapeutic grade oil. There is
electricity and life force, too.

Since the healing oils of wintergreen and birch are
chemically more than 85% methyl salicylate, there are
some places, such as in England, where pure synthetic methyl salicylate is sold and labeled as if it were natural wintergreen. A chemist, with all his or her equipment, may not be able to determine the difference
between the natural and the laboratory produced products, but the discerning powers of the human body can
tell the two apart instantly and reacts accordingly.

Synthetically produced methyl salicylate is toxic,
while its naturally grown cousin is not. In addition to
being non-toxic, the natural product also has curative

powers while its artificial counterpart does not.

Some aromatherapists don't understand this and decline to use wintergreen or birch oils for any purpose. They are especially alarmed at the idea of applying these oils neat, as is done in raindrop technique. What they don't realize is that the toxicities they may have experienced or read of do not exist with true therapeutic grade oils, only with synthetic or adulterated grades.

For more information see *The Chemistry of Essential Oils Made Simple.* (pp. 324) This book has a whole section entitled "Beyond Chemistry."

The Cleverness of Counterfeiting Chemists

Because the profits are so high in selling cheap-to-produce non-therapeutic oils at costly-to-produce therapeutic prices, the temptation to do so has created many laboratories and teams of chemists who are very skillful in imitating the chemical composition of natural oils. Many of these are in France, with a reputation where excellent therapeutic grade oils can be obtained. Some unscrupulous French businesses bottle cheap adulterated imitations in containers saying "Made in France," producing them for export only, knowing that they would never pass the rigorous French standards in a government testing lab. Some counterfeit oils are so carefully compounded they are virtually impossible to detect, even with the most sophisticated laboratory equipment.

What some chemists do is to synthetically combine the ten or fifteen most abundant ingredients contained in a natural oil, which are the ones the testing lab will measure to see if the proportions are right. But a natural oil contains hundreds of components, most in trace amounts and most, as yet, of undetermined composition. Testing labs do not and cannot test for every component because it would be economically prohibitive and, at this time, scientifically impossible. The counterfeit companies know this and take advantage of it.

Hence, when an authentic oil and a false oil are tested for their most abundant constituents, they can both look identical insofar as the analysis was taken. But the imitation oil will have no healing capability because it is dead. It would be like assembling all of the major parts of a cat in perfect form and expecting it to perform as a real cat. The same amounts of hair, bone, skin and tissue may be there, but there is no life. Only God can give that.

While the laboratory cannot always tell the difference between bad and good oils, humans can tell the difference right away. Either the oils render benefits, or they don't. An electromagnetic frequency measurement would also reveal the truth, but chemical laboratories, thus far, are not equipped for routine measurements of electromagnetic frequencies in the megahertz and nanovolt range, as would be necessary.

Dr. Herve Casabianca (Ph.D.), Director of the the largest essential oils testing laboratory in France and chairman of the International Standards Organization committee on oils, has come to the conclusion that the only way one can be certain that they are obtaining true therapeutic grade oils is to "Know your grower. Know your distiller. And know your supplier. Otherwise," he says, "the chemists have become so clever that they can sometimes fool even the best of laboratories."

The bottom line is that one cannot absolutely confirm the authenticity of an oil by a gas chromatogram, a mass spectrogram, or by any other chemical analytic technique available to modern science. It takes human experience with the oil to determine that. And who wants to be a guinea pig? You want to receive and administer real healing oils, and nothing else, without going through trial and error.

It Takes Life to Produce Life

It takes a life process to produce a living substance. Only God can do that. Chemistry is not all there is to the components of an essential oil. There is also electromagnetic frequency, or life force. If frequency is measured, you find that synthetically produced substances are motionless and inert. Zero frequency. At the same time, a naturally grown component in an intact oil gently coaxed from the plant with all of its companion components is vibrant and full of vigor, eager to heal and administer therapy. In fact, there is intelligence in essential oils that have been properly grown and extracted without adulteration. Oils produced by living processes are living. Oils produced by mechanical man-made processes are lifeless.

Only God can make a therapeutic oil. All we can do is to extract it as lovingly as possible and leave it untouched. It is man's arrogance that makes him think he can improve on nature by tampering with the oil. Essential oils are God's gift to everyone. They can never be copyrighted or trademarked or patented for profit. Anyone with the patience and willingness can learn to produce them or to find producers they can trust. Their applications, while healing, are not the practice of medicine. In the Biblical tradition, the application of essential oils was the practice of religion. Every American has the right to exercise that freedom.

Obtaining Oils that Heal

Where can healing oils of Biblical quality be obtained? The major oils discussed in this book are commercially available from one or more sources. There are a number of growers and distilleries in North Amreica that produce high quality oils fulfilling all of the criteria for therapeutic grade.

Look for the designation "AFNOR" or AFNOR-EC" on the label. Oils that carry this fulfill European standards for essential oils. (There are no American standards as yet, but they are currently in the making.) AFNOR stands for "Association Francaise de Normalization." It is a French government-approved organization under the administrative supervision of the French Ministry for Industry. EC stands for "European Commission." Oils that meet this standard must regularly send samples to France for testing before they can print "AFNOR" on their labels. The ISO (International Standardization Organization) in Geneva, Switzerland, is a worldwide federation of national standards bodies drawn from 130 countries. The ISO has adopted the AFNOR standards for essential oils as the international standard.

There is only one North American company that routinely sends oil samples abroad for AFNOR testing and that is Young Living Essential Oils, Inc., (YLEO) a network marketing company. In addition to meeting AFNOR standards, therapeutic grade oils must also be organically grown, unadulterated, properly distilled, and meet other criteria which YLEO oils do. Inquire to see if there is a Young Living distributor in your neighborhood, perhaps a relative or someone you know, from whom you may purchase Biblical grade oils. You may also purchase Biblical grade oils from the internet at <bibleoils.younglivingworld.com> (There is no "www" in front of this address.)

The AFNOR designation applies only to single oils. European testing laboratories do not test blends. Blends of oils do not carry this designation even when all of the ingredients meet AFNOR standards. If all of the single oils carried by a company meet therapeutic standards, then you can safely assume that all of that company's blends do, too. Therapeutic grade oils are not usually sold in retail stores.

Over 90% of the oils sold as "essential" in America are food or fragrance grades and unsuitable for healing applications. So one cannot go just anywhere and expect to find therapeutic grade oils. One has to search and be discerning in one's search. One must also educate oneself thoroughly in the use and application of essential oils to gain their full benefits. Be discriminating in what you read. There are false teachings out there as well as fake oils. Some of the general references on oils, aromatherapy, and related topics that we recommend are starred with asterisks in the bibliography (pp. 300-304) with their titles in bold-faced type.

Chapter 14
A Bible Oils Program You Can Do

A new concept has been developed that is working well. It's fun. It's easy. And you can do it. It is a scriptural oils program that can be done in living rooms, churches, community centers, schools, and other public places. It is an opportunity for you to provide a unique and valuable service to your community. The program also works quite well as a one-on-one presentation with a single person, a couple, or small group around a kitchen table. It appeals to a whole segment of society who might otherwise never come into contact with the concept of healing oils. This program offers a great opportunity for people to learn of the wonderful healing miracles possible through essential oils.

What you do is schedule a program entitled "HEALING OILS OF THE *BIBLE*." You don't have to be an expert on oils or an authority on *Bible* scripture to do this. This book contains all the background information you need, and much more. The instructions in this chapter, plus the handouts you can photocopy from Appendices E and F, make it possible for anyone who can read to do this program and do it well. All you need is this book. If someone stumps you with a question during your presentation, just refer them to this publication saying, "It's in the book."

Churches are particularly appropriate places to offer this program. We have found churches receptive to the idea. When seeking permission to offer the program, give the pastor a copy of the program notes (Photocopies of Appendices E and F, pp. 276-299) and the brochure on "Twelve Oils of Ancient Scripture." Also show them a Scriptural Oils Kit and let them smell the Frankincense or the Sandalwood or one of the other oils in which they may express an interest. You should also show them this book, either loaning them a copy or giving them a copy. That always opens doors.

We have found that churches are not only willing to provide the facilities for the meeting, but will put it in their bulletins, newsletters, and on the church calendar. Some will even make a special announcement to the congregation in church. I tell the pastor that I will put some posters around town, place an article in the local newspaper, and publicize the event in various ways. Most churches look upon this as outreach and like the idea of attracting new people to come to a program on their grounds who are not already members of their congregations. We encourage everyone coming to bring their *Bibles*.

As for the program, itself, we build it upon the Twelve Oils of Ancient Scripture Kit™, but we also use Joy™, Exodus II™, Thieves™, 3 Wise Men™, Valor™, and sometimes the 7th Heaven Kit™. All of these blends and kits contain Biblical oils. We pass around the bottles of oils as we talk and take turns reading the appropriate scriptures from the *Bible*. Sharing the oils is the most important part of the program. What you say is secondary.

Always Start with Joy

We open the program by passing around the oil of Joy™. The *Bible* mentions oils of joy, gladness, or rejoicing in Isaiah 61:3, Psalms 45:7-8, Proverbs 27:9 and Hebrews 1:9. Before the program starts, I find four people with their *Bibles* who will have these verses ready to read when the time comes.

We finish up with Spikenard, which is mentioned in the *Bible* seven times and was the last oil received by Christ before going to the cross. We ask the group: "When Jesus was anointed with Spikenard just before his arrest and crucifixion, was it on his feet or on his head?" We take a poll. Some will say head. Some feet. We have four people selected in advance who are willing to read these four passages. We read them in this order: First Matthew 26:6-7, then Luke 7:36-38, then Mark 14:3, and last of all John 12:1-3. What we discover, along with the audience, is that the four scriptures present more than one version of what appears at first to be the same incident in the life of Christ. (An explanation and resolution of the apparent contradictions is contained in Chapter 10 in the section subtitled "The Mystery of the Anointing Woman.")

We close with Mark 6:12-13: "And they went out . . . and they anointed with oil many that were sick and healed them." After reading this scripture, we conclude the program saying words like: "Those of us who use, administer, and teach the use of these oils feel that we are carrying on the work of Jesus as taught to his disciples and as expressed in this passage from Mark . . .etc."

The programs have all been extremely well received, and everyone wants to do it again. Once, when we did it in St. Louis, we put a couple of announcements in widely read municipal publications and got so many calls that our facilities were too small. For almost half of those who called in advance to reserve a place, we had to take their name and number and tell them that this session was full and that we'd let them know the next time we planned to do a *Bible* Oils Program.

Healings on the Spot

We have found that after passing around more than a dozen of these spiritually uplifting oils, by the end of the program, people are so excited and happy they don't want to leave. It's like being in "Seventh Heaven," said one participant. One lady came with a splitting headache, and by the time we had passed the first two or three oils around, she was headache free and felt great. Six months after we did one program, a lady who had attended reported that her allergies had disappeared during the program that very night and that she had not needed her allergy medications ever since. Another attendee who had been taking Sudefed® for sinus congestion twice a day for fifteen years. His sinuses cleared up that night. He now carries peppermint oil with him at all times and hasn't taken Sudefed since. It is also common for those suffering from arthritis pain to receive relief as the oils are passed around. Others coming down with the flu, a cold or a sore throat have their immunities restored during the program and never get the sickness they feared was upon them.

The program normally takes two-and-a-half hours. After one of our presentations, which was from 7:00 to 9:30 P.M. (with about 20 people present), no one left for over an hour afterwards and the whole room was buzzing with everyone talking with each other. Some were so thrilled by the information and by what the oils had done for them they stayed until nearly midnight.

A Complete Set of Notes for You

Appendices E and F serve as a complete outline and set of notes for the presenter, which also serve as a handout to the participants. Permission is granted on page 276 to photocopy as many copies as you need for your programs. You don't have to be a theologian or a trained aromatherapist. With this book and those notes, you have everything you need by way of information.

The success of this idea has exceeded our expectations. It has turned out to be one of the most enjoyable things we have ever done. The notes are designed so that you can tailor them to your needs to make the program as long or as short as you wish. When doing the program, take a set of the notes you will be handing out to your audience and scribble notes to yourself of the comments you want to make and where to interject them as you go.

Publicity is Key

In publicizing your program, make up posters to place in churches and public places around town. Also mail out copies of your poster or flyer to every radio, TV station, newspaper, and church in your area. Use the Yellow pages to get the addresses. If in a church or public facility, the program would normally be free. If given elsewhere, you may charge a fee. When there is a charge, we normally allow children and teens in free.

If the program is without charge, you can obtain free publicity via the media as a public service announcement. The media usually requires a phone contact before they will make a public service announcement or list it in the community church calendar. In this case, emphasize that it is FREE and OPEN TO THE PUBLIC.

Your poster should always have the time, date, day of the week, and address of the program, as well as a person's name with their phone number as a contact. Also include whether it is free or for a fee.

A sample of how the poster copy can read is given on the next page. Use brightly colored papers. Distribute lots of them. You can never have too many posters. It takes time, but two or three hours putting up posters around town will definitely pay off.

Purpose of the Program

The primary purpose is public education on the topic of HEALING OILS OF THE *BIBLE*. Most people do not know the important role that essential oils played in the lives of Biblical people, nor do they know about the healing power of the oils. This a good program to offer to churches and schools. It can also be done in living rooms, libraries, and other meeting places. It can be used as an effective way to interest people in learning more about the benefits of the oils and using them on themselves and their families.

Time for the Program

Set aside two-and-a-half hours for the program, including a short break half way through. If you include the Seventh Heaven kit, plan for another 15 minutes. The Seventh Heaven part (Appendix E) is optional and usually omitted when making a presentation in a home or for a couple around the dining room table.

Plan at least an hour's slack time afterwards for people to linger, enjoy the oils, and talk.

Shorter versions of the program can be arranged by omitting parts and letting participants read the literature you hand out.

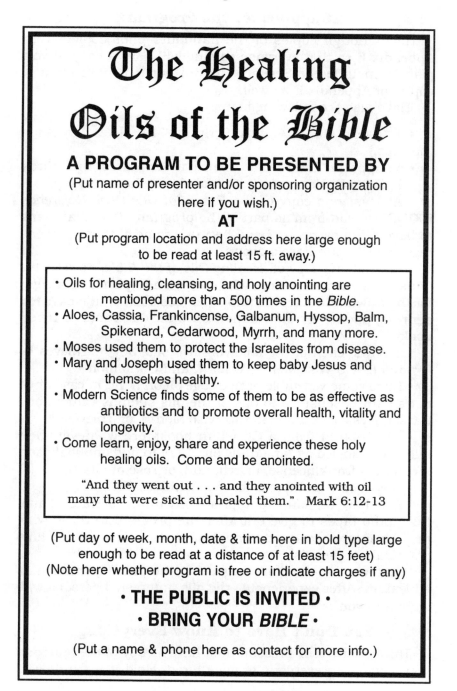

The Healing
Oils of the Bible

A PROGRAM TO BE PRESENTED BY
(Put name of presenter and/or sponsoring organization
here if you wish.)
AT
(Put program location and address here large enough
to be read at least 15 ft. away.)

- Oils for healing, cleansing, and holy anointing are
    mentioned more than 500 times in the *Bible*.
- Aloes, Cassia, Frankincense, Galbanum, Hyssop, Balm,
    Spikenard, Cedarwood, Myrrh, and many more.
- Moses used them to protect the Israelites from disease.
- Mary and Joseph used them to keep baby Jesus and
    themselves healthy.
- Modern Science finds some of them to be as effective as
    antibiotics and to promote overall health, vitality and
    longevity.
- Come learn, enjoy, share and experience these holy
    healing oils. Come and be anointed.

"And they went out . . . and they anointed with oil
many that were sick and healed them."   Mark 6:12-13

(Put day of week, month, date & time here in bold type large
enough to be read at a distance of at least 15 feet)
(Note here whether program is free or indicate charges if any)

· THE PUBLIC IS INVITED ·
· BRING YOUR *BIBLE* ·

(Put a name & phone here as contact for more info.)

Supplies for the Program

Have enough copies of the handouts photocopied from Appendix F so that everyone coming will have a copy. If you plan to include the Seventh Heaven portion, have enough copies of Appendix E as well.

Have also the following items.

• 1 "Twelve Oils of Ancient Scripture" Kit. (Get labels for the caps.)

• A supply of "Twelve Oils of Ancient Scriptures" Brochures

• 1 "Seventh Heaven" Kit (Get labels for the caps.)

• At least one copy of the *Essential Oils Desk Reference* (EODR) to read from as part of the program. (You may want to have a few extras on hand because some of those present may want to purchase a copy)

• At least one copy of, *Healing Oils of the Bible*, to refer to. (Plus a few extras for those who may wish to purchase a copy for their own.) Contact the publisher (see back of title page for address/phone) for information on bulk discounts of these books.

• 1 bottle each of the following five oils: Joy™, Thieves™, Exodus II™, 3 Wise Men™, Valor™, and Cinnamon.

• Have some vegetable or massage oil on hand in case anyone's skin is sensitive to one of the oils such as Cinnamon, Cassia, Hyssop, Exodus II™, 3 Wise Men™, or Thieves™.

• Also obtain from a Christian bookstore whatever they may have labeled as "anointing oils." Try to find one that says it contains frankincense, myrrh, and/or rose of sharon.

• Have some toothpicks for the Onycha

• Also have on hand appropriate brochures, literature, and free audio tapes to give out after the program to those who may be interested in additional information on the healing potentials of the oils.

Whatever you do, don't forget that the primary mission is education. After experiencing the oils, interested persons will approach you.

You Don't Have to Know Everything

Throughout your presentation, have a copy of the handout you have given everyone in your hand. Hold it up and read from it. Have others read most of the *Bible* passages as you carry out the program. Don't feel like you have to memorize anything. Relax and enjoy the program along with your guests, letting them be a part of it.

Let the oils make the presentation. They can speak for themselves. If people want more information, they can read the materials you have provided them later and at their own pace.

If people want to give spontaneous testimonies, I usually let them do it, but only to a point. This is a quasi-religious meeting, not a scientific one, and participants may have great stories to tell. True healing is a religious experience. As group leader you have to be sure that you can finish the program on time. When good testimonies are being told I allow it and sometimes cut short what I have to say so we don't run over-time At the same time, you have valuable information to present, also. So use your discretion in allowing testimonies.

Set-Up for the Program

The program is best done in small enough groups where everyone can sit in a circle facing everybody else and where oils can be easily passed around. Large living rooms or church Sunday School rooms are perfect. Dining room or kitchen tables are ideal, too. Encourage people to bring a *Bible*. Have name tags where people write their first names in large print. A medium-tipped felt marker works well and can be read at least 10-15 feet away.

Remember the success of your program will be measured by the extent to which everyone feels that they were active participants. When the program is well done, people will be energized, inspired, and won't want to leave. Most will desire to stay and enjoy the uplifting spirit, exhilaration, and fellowship that experiencing these oils as a group will generate.

Program Outline

1. As people arrive, pass out copies of the handouts, along with a copy of the brochure on "Twelve Oils of Ancient Scriptures." Have them sign in on a sheet giving their names, addresses, phone numbers, and any other information you deem of interest for followup purposes. See that everyone has a legible name tag.

2. Before the program begins, have all the scriptures you plan to have read on little slips of paper. Pass them to people who have brought a *Bible* who are willing to read out loud. There will be 24 *Bible* passages read during the program (6 for you to read as the leader and 18 by others). Some people may read several verses. If you wish, just put the slips of paper in a hat and let people draw. Make it fun. Then tell them to use the slips to mark each passage in their *Bible*s and that you will call on them when the time comes for those verses in the program.

Verses the leader should read are: Proverbs 21:30; Numbers 16:46-50; Isaiah 59: 20; 60:3, 6; Psalms 51:1-4, 7; Mark 6:7, 10-13; and James 5:14. Mark these on your copy of the notes so you will know when they should be read in the program.

The 18 verses to be put on slips of paper and distributed to others to read are as follows:

Exodus 30:22-31	Psalms 45:7-8
Proverbs 27:9	Isaiah 61:3
Hebrews 1:9	John 19:39
Matthew 2:11	Exodus 30:34-36
Exodus 12:22	Psalms 51:7
John 19:29	Esther 2:12
Mark 15:23	Esther 2:7
Matthew 26:6-7	Luke 7:36-38
Mark 14:3	John 12:1-3

Also choose two people to read from the *Essential Oils Desk Reference*, 2nd edition, (EODR) pages 96 and 124 on Exodus II and 3 Wise Men, respectively.

3. When the time comes to start, be punctual. If it is in a church, request the pastor or other appropriate person to open with a prayer. Go around the room and have everyone introduce themselves asking them to mention if they have had any experience with essential oils? A brief testimony or two here is okay, but don't let it get too drawn out. There's lots of material to cover in the program. You won't have time for this if the group is too large, i.e. if more than 20-25 people.

4. Have everyone go to the first page of the notes and you, as the leader, read or summarize the items at the top starting with the brief scripture **Proverbs 21:20**. Mention that essen-

tial oils are detoxifying, even when inhaled, which is the first step toward healing. **Emphasize that everyone attending the program needs to drink plenty of water** so that the loosened toxins can flush from the body through normal channels and not be reabsorbed or cause discomfort.

5. At this time in the program you need to briefly make four points:

(i) Mention how the fragrances of essential oils were in the Garden of Eden and what implications that has for us today. (see Chapter One, pp. 1-2.)

(ii) Explain the two types of oils plants make, essential and fatty. (see Chapter 2, pp. 22-23)

(iii) Comment on how the original healers were priests who often did their healing in temples, and how that relates to today. (See Chapter Three.)

(iv) Explain the Biblical meaning of "anoint," which is to "rub or massage." Point out the similarity in meaning and pronunciation between the Hebrew word for anoint "masach," the English word "massage." (See Chapter Four, pp. 58-61)

(v) At this point I like to demonstrate a true Biblical anointing. Either choose a person to whom you feel guided or ask for a volunteer, explaining that you may mess up their hair. Then choose a Biblical oil with a strong fragrance, like frankincense, spikenard, cedarwood, or 3 Wise Men™. I usually take out the dropper cap and pour a little on the top of their head. (Be careful not to pour too close to the forehead because you don't want oil to run into their eyes. If such an accident should occur, immediately have them tilt their face up and have them pour some vegetable oil into their eyes. No harm will come, should this happen. Only temporary discomfort.) Assuming no oils got into the eyes, mention that in Psalm 133:2 Moses poured precious oils upon the head of Aaron until it ran down his beard and down to the skirts of his garments, but assure the chosen receiver that you won't be using that much oil in this instance. After a generous amount of oil has been poured on the crown of the head, then massage it into the scalp, around the ears, around the neck and shoulders in a loving manner and verbally give them a blessing. This is a true anointing in the Biblical sense, a pouring on of the oil accompanied by a prayer of blessing and a loving touch. If anyone questions your authority to anoint in the name of the Lord, simply refer them to I Peter 2:5 & 9, saying that you have been authorized by the Word of God. You will often find that the person chosen for the anointing at that particular meeting was picked by God and their lives are blessed from that moment forward in a special way.

6.   Have four people to look up and read: **Psalms 45:7-8**, **Proverbs 27:9**, **Isaiah 61:3**, and **Hebrews 1:9**, referring either to the "Oil of Joy" or "Oil of Gladness," or to the fact that "Ointments rejoice the heart." Point out the Biblical implication of associating an oil with an emotion. (See Chapter Six.)

Hold up the oil blend of JOY, explaining that it contains rose oil, with a frequency of 320 Megahertz, the highest frequency of any known substance and a scent often reported to accompany spiritual visions and miracles. (See Chapter Eight.)

Explain that some people taking antidepressant drugs have found JOY to be mood elevating and have been able to reduce their dependence upon pharmaceuticals by diffusing JOY, rubbing it on their bodies, and/or inhaling it.

7. **DEMONSTRATE** how to put a drop of oil in the palm, make several clockwise circles with your fingers, rub your palms together and cup them over your nose and mouth (avoiding the eyes) inhaling the vapors. Request that they respect the precious oils being passed around, trying to avoid getting the oil on the outside of the bottles, and taking only a drop. If you prefer not to pass around the actual bottles of oil, you can take small pieces of paper about two inches square, print the name of the oil on the paper, and, put a drop of the designated oil on the paper. You can pass that around instead of the actual oil. People can still inhale the fragrance from this. Personally, I like to pass the bottles, but sometimes I do half and half, partly passing bottles and partly pass-

ing perfumed papers. At this point in the program, **PASS AROUND THE OIL OF JOY**.

8. As Joy is circulating the room, take this opportunity to explain how the nose is wired differently than the other four senses and that it carries molecules directly into the emotional center of the brain where traumatic memories are stored and that essential oils are a vehicle by which repressed emotions can be released. (See Chapter Two, sections on emotions, and Chapter Six for this information.)

Also at this time, mention that there are 33 species of essential oils and aromatic plants mentioned in the *Bible* and choose a statement at the end of Chapter Five to read as a statement of how many times they are mentioned in the *Bible*. The statement I read is the last one that says there are "1,015 references." You need to have read all of Chapter Five if you say this so you will understand where that number came from. Comment that every time the *Bible* used words or phrases such as anointing oil, incense, ointment, spices, perfumes, odors, or sweet savors, aromas, or fragrances that essential oils are always implied. Mention that natural oils were the only fragrances available in Biblical times, the synthetic ones of today having not yet been invented.

9. Before going to the next page of *Bible* Oils Notes, point out that the 14 principal Biblical aromatic oils listed at the beginning of the notes all contain phenols or phenylpropanoids, sesquiterpenes, and/or monoterpenes, and that most of the oils contain all three of these classes of compounds. Learn to pronounce these three words (the strong syllables are underlined):

Fee . nal. <u>Pro</u> . pa. noids
<u>Ses</u> . qui. <u>Ter</u> . pens
<u>Mah</u> . no . <u>Ter</u> . pens

Then explain that these three constituents are unique to

essential oils and when produced naturally by the plant have the intelligence and capability of cleansing the receptor sites of our cells (phenols), erasing incorrect information in the DNA or cellular memory (sesquiterpenes), and reprogramming God's original plan (correct information) into the cellular intelligence (monoterpenes). In this way, essential oils can actually correct the cause of a disease at the cellular level and facilitate a permanent, and, sometimes, instantaneous healing. However, emphasize that oils react differently to every person and that no claims can be made as to what oils may or may not do in any particular instance. (See Chapter Two, section on "A Quick Course on Chemistry" for this information.)

10. Have everyone turn to page 280 of the notes listing Exodus II and 3 Wise Men. Note that all the ingredients except Spikenard are mentioned in the Book of Exodus. Have someone read from comments on Exodus II in the second edition of the *Essential Oils Desk Reference* (**EODR), page 96**, first paragraph only down to last sentence, "This blend was designed. . ."). Then **PASS AROUND EXODUS II.** Suggest rubbing some on the forehead. Explain what this passage implies with respect to the transient value of antibiotics versus the timeless value of essential oils. (See Chapter Four, section on "Oils vs. Antibiotics.")

As an optional part of the program you can point out that the blend, Thieves, has similar antiseptic properties to Exodus II, explaining how Thieves got its name. (See Chapter Four, section entitled 'Immune to the Black Plague.") **PASS AROUND THIEVES.**

11. Have someone read the **EODR, page 124**, the short paragraph under 3 Wise Men noting that all of the individual oils of this blend are known to help in the releasing and resolution of deep-seated trauma and repressed emotions. **PASS AROUND 3 WISE MEN**. Suggest rubbing some on the temples.

As an optional part of the program, point out that all of the oils in 3 Wise Men are mentioned in the *Bible* except spruce, which was an oil used in Biblical times, but not mentioned.

In particular, mention that the Roman soldiers used some of the oils in 3 Wise Men, such as spruce, because they had the emotional impact of giving them courage. Tell how the soldiers would rub oils on their feet and shoulders or just inhale them before battle to give them courage. With such courage and such oils, they conquered the known world of their day. A blend of oils such as this is VALOR, whose first ingredient is spruce. Valor also contains frankincense. (See Chapter Four, section on "Anointments for Courage and Spiritual Awakening" for more on this.)

PASS AROUND VALOR. Encourage people to rub it on their necks. Tell them that this oil is used in raindrop technique and has the property of stimulating one's spine to self-adjust. Ask people to note if their spine moves when inhaling or anointing themselves with this oil. Sometimes spines snap into place as people sit during the program.

12. If you include the 7th Heaven Kit in your program, have everyone turn to the pages you have handed to them on this and explain to them the origin of the phrase. (See Appendix E for this information.) Read **II Corinthians 12:2, 4** quoted at the top of the notes on the 7th Heaven Kit. EXPLAIN that it was a common belief and concept among the Jews in Christ's day that saintly individuals could be described as to their level of spirituality according to "Levels of Heaven" experienced in their personal communications, prayers, and meditations with God. The *Bible* does not expound on this point because it would have been understood by most Jews in Jesus' time without any comment. People hearing Paul's reference to the Third Heaven would have known exactly what he was talking about. According to this Jewish concept, the highest level of spiritual perception, divine ecstasy, holy communion, or union with God is, of course, "Seventh Heaven."

13. Point out that the 7th Heaven Kit contains seven oil blends specifically formulated for spiritual upliftment. All of these blends contain Biblical oils which were used for spiritually elevating purposes in Biblical times. NOTE that three of the four oils of the world containing the highest

known concentration of sesquiterpenes are Biblical (Cedarwood, Spikenard, and Sandalwood). Sesquiterpenes carry oxygen to the brain and stimulate the pineal and pituitary glands. These oils have been reported to stimulate positive emotional states. **THEN SIMPLY PASS AROUND EACH OF THE SEVEN OILS WITHOUT COMMENTARY. Move immediately to the next section** of the notes, mentioning that an in-depth discussion of the oils of this kit and all the other oils can be found in the EODR and that you have a few copies that can be purchased if anyone wishes.

14. On the remaining pages of the notes, fourteen oils of the *Bible* are listed with notes—the twelve in the Scriptural Oils Kit plus Cinnamon and Calamus. As you come to each oil, select a point or two from the notes that are interesting to you, but don't try to cover all the material. It would take many hours to do that. Interested parties can read the complete notes on their own afterwards or buy the book, *Healing Oils of the Bible*. The most important part is to **PASS EACH OIL AROUND** as you come to it. Caution them that some of them may be irritating to the skin, like Cinnamon, Cassia, and Hyssop. All of the oils are safe to put on the palm, but some would be better not rubbed elsewhere where the skin is more sensitive. People can be their own judge on this. Mention that you do have some mixing oil on hand if needed, and that if anyone's skin starts to heat up or get red, you can cool it off immediately with the vegetable oil you have on hand. As an alternative to passing the actual bottles of oil around, you can write the names of the oils on slips of paper placing a drop of the oil on the surface. Passing around scented papers avoids any possibility of someone reacting adversely to the oils. Personally, I like to pass the bottles for most of the oils and have had no problems in doing it this way.

15. As you come to each oil have participants look up the scriptures selected in bold-faced type and have your

designated people read them aloud. There are too many scriptural references to oils to read all of them mentioned on the handouts. (See Appendix C.) Those in bold will be enough for the program. Involve as many different people as you can in these readings.

AS EACH OIL IS DISCUSSED, PASS IT AROUND.

16. **Comments to Make:** The comments given below are suggestions only. They are what I might say in doing this program. Say whatever is natural and of interest to you and don't worry what you leave out. No one will know but you. Besides, your audience will have a pile of notes to study when they get home and if they really want more info they can read this book. Try to keep your program to no more than 2.0-2.5 hours. The information of this book is for background only, not all to be presented. 2.5 hours worth of content is about all anyone will want to hear at one time. Besides, the most important part of the program is sharing the oils. Oils can speak for themselves.

Scriptures to Read and Suggested Comments to Make While Passing Around the Oils

A. **ALOES/SANDALWOOD: Read John 19:39** (Jesus' burial oils) Note: 75-100 lbs of aloes and myrrh would be worth $150.000–$200.000 in today's market. The incredible value of these spices demonstrates two things:

(a) The wealth of Nicodemus and Joseph of Arimathea must have been incredibly great and

(b) Their respect and reverence for their Lord and Savior must also have been very great.

B. **CASSIA & CINNAMON:** Cassia and Cinnamon are in God's Holy anointing oil described in the scripture already read, Exodus 30: 22-31) Point out the similarity in fragrance of these two oils. Note that they are actually two species of the same genus, *Cinnamomum*, and that they are in the Laurel family of plants, along with Bay, another oil of Biblical times. Suggest that people put a little on their palms, but to only inhale these two, inasmuch as they can be caustic and irritating to the more sensitive areas of our skin. Have some mixing oil on hand just in case someone rubs it on their face or arms. Point out that these oils are extremely effective in fighting bacteria and viruses. They protected the Israelites from disease. They can also support our immune systems against colds and flu's simply by inhaling them or putting them on the soles of our feet.

C. **CEDARWOOD:** Pass around with selected comments from the notes. Skip the reading of scriptures on this oil. Point out that Cedarwood may have been the first oil to be obtained by distillation, inasmuch as the Egyptians and Sumerians were doing it over 5,000 years ago, using it for embalming, for ritual purposes, as a disinfectant and for other medicinal purposes. Point out that in Leviticus 14 there is a cleansing ritual for leprosy where cedarwood and hyssop oils are used and applied to the tip or top of the right ear, the right thumb, and the right toe. In reflexology and emotional release, that portion of the ear is where one releases and resolves issues regarding their parents. The thumb and big toe are the trigger points for clearing fears of the unknown and mental blocks against learning, while the big toe is a point for clearing addictions and compulsive behavior. The scent of cedarwood can help clear many buried emotions, including feelings of pride or conceit. Hyssop (which we will discuss later) is a releaser of swallowed emotions and a spiritual cleanser of past sin and immorality. (See Chapter 3, the section entitled "Did Biblical Priests Know Reflexology?")

Point out that among the aspects of cedarwood, it is an insect repellent. Ask the audience how many of them have cedar chests or cedar closets or cedar drawers? Ask them why? To repel moths, they will say. The oil is in the wood and the scent stays in the furniture indefinitely, for the life of the wood.

Mention that Solomon built his temple and palace out of the Cedars of Lebanon. (See Chapter Nine.) Thus, his places to live, govern, and worship all had the vapors of cedarwood oil in the air. Cedarwood oil contains the highest concentration of sesquiterpenes of any known substance (98%).

Sesquiterpenes oxygenate the brain and support clear thinking, which is what wise rulers need to have. Perhaps King Solomon was wiser than we thought. Perhaps he knew of the aromatherapeutic benefits of cedar and applied that knowledge in building his palace and temple.

D. **CYPRESS:**   Pass around with selected comments from the notes. Skip the reading of scriptures for the oil of Cypress. Comment that it is supportive of the immune and cardiovascular systems and is rich in monoterpenes.

E. **GALBANUM**   **Read Exodus 30:34-36**

Four oils are mentioned in this passage: Galbanum, Stacte, Frankincense, and Onycha. Start with Galbanum. As you pass it around, mention that Galbanum is in the parsley family and has an earthy, parsley-like smell that is emotionally grounding.

Then talk briefly about Stacte. Stacte (pronounced 'stack-tee') is another name for Myrrh. Myrrh is the only oil that is an ingredient in both the holy anointing oil and the holy incense. (See Exodus 30:23, 34) Why would God mandate myrrh in both formulas? Answer: Myrrh is the most commonly used fixing oil of ancient times. Fixing oils are combined with other fragrances to make them last longer. Myrrh is one of the best oils in the world for this purpose.

One could say that it appears that God was knowledgeable in aromatherapy and the science of creating blends with lasting fragrances. On the other hand, God is omniscient, knowing everything including all about aromatherapy. In fact, God is the origin and source of all wisdom. Man merely rediscovers truth created by God. This is why we call God "The First Aromatherapist" in Chapter One.

Mention that by God's command: (1) the holy incense was to be burned in the tabernacle or temple twenty-four hours a day; (2) the "apothecaries and perfumers" mentioned in the *Bible* who compounded the fragrances for worship were the Levite priests. (3) Creating blends of oils for worship, as well as for medicine, was one of their priestly duties.

Sirach, a book in the *Old Testament Apocrypha*, was written around 180 B.C. (See Appendix B) The formula for holy incense given in Exodus 30:34 is also found in Sirach 24:15. Thus, more than 1,000 years after Moses was given the formula by God, it was still used in Jewish worship and continued to be used through the time of Christ.

F. **FRANKINCENSE:** Mention that Egyptian tradition considered frankincense to be a universal cure-all. One bit of wisdom gleaned from Egyptian antiquity says that "frankincense is good for everything from gout to a broken head." That would be the Egyptian way of saying "good for everything from head to toe." —

Leader **Read Numbers 16:46-50.** (Aaron stops a plague.) Point out that the incense used by Aaron is the holy incense of Exodus 30:34-36, which was just read, containing Galbanum, Myrrh, Onycha, and Frankincense. Point out that fumigation was one of the ways that Biblical people made use of essential oils. (See Chapter Twelve.)

Then the leader should read the verses from Isaiah which prophesy the gifts of the 3 wise men (Leader **Read Isaiah 59:20, 60:3, 6.)** Note that the Hebrew word translated into English as "incense" in this passage is "lebonah" which is Frankincense. There are five other places in the *Bible* where lebonah was translated as "incense" when, in fact, it should have been Frankincense. (See Table 3-A, Appendix A.) These verses are considered to be a prophecy of the coming of Jesus and the visit of the three wise men.

Then have someone **Read Matthew 2:11.** (gifts of the wise men). Point out that Frankincense is okay to inhale, rub on the skin, and also to take internally. The Israelites used it all three ways.

Mention that Mary and Joseph would have appreciated this gift as the anointing oil for newborn sons of kings. They would have rubbed it all over the tiny body of their Christ child. They would also have understood that this oil is a healing oil good for almost anything from cuts and bruises to the common cold. Hence, they would have understood it as a gift for them to use throughout the infancy of Jesus to help protect him and keep him strong and healthy. The wise men would not have to explain these things to Mary and Joseph because they would have already been familiar with the uses of frankincense, as were most people in Biblical times. This is why Matthew does not bother to elaborate on the applications of these oils in his Gospel. He did not foresee that 2,000 years later westerners, having no experience with healing oils, would be uninformed in such matters.

Comment that frankincense has been diffused or burned in Catholic churches for centuries and still is. Frankincense is also in many perfumes and colognes, including the best selling men's fragrance, Old Spice®.

G. **HYSSOP:** **Read Exodus 12:22.** In this passage of Exodus Moses asked the elders of Israel to sacrifice a lamb and use a branch of hyssop to apply the blood of the lamb to the door posts of their dwellings. This was the first Passover. The spirit of death was to pass through Egypt that night, killing all the firstborn sons of every household except those marked with the blood of the lamb from the hyssop branch. While the symbology of the blood of the lamb saving the sons of the Israelites has strong significance for Christians it is also interesting to note that the ancient Hebrews also believed that the scent of hyssop would repel evil spirits. God's instructions were to "strike" the lintel and door posts, which would have bruised the hyssop leaves and released the scent of its oil. (See Chapter 12.) Thus, the fragrance of the hyssop was a part of the ritual to cause the evil spirit of death to pass over the Israelites that night.

Read Psalm 51:7. Comment that the fragrance of hyssop was considered to be spiritually purifying and an aid in cleansing oneself from sin, immorality, evil thoughts, or bad habits. Ask why the psalmist, in this case, would say "purge me with hyssop?" The leader should then read the beginning of **Psalm 51:1-4, 7**, pointing out that the prelude to this Psalm says, ". . . A Psalm of David, when Nathan the prophet came unto him, after he had gone in to Bathsheba." (II Samuel 12:1-14) David had committed adultery and murder and seemed to have no conscience about it. As King he had thought himself above the law and the commandments. Then Nathan came and opened his eyes to the gravity of his transgressions. This Psalm was written during David's grief in his realization of the magnitude of his terrible actions.

The calling for hyssop oil (inhaled and applied to the body) to purge oneself from iniquity has a scientific basis. Hyssop is about 50% ketones, which act like phenols and cleanse receptor sites. Hyssop also contains 5–10% sesquiterpenes that delete addictions, compulsions, and other ungodly directives from the DNA. Hyssop is also 20-30% monoterpenes which reprogram the DNA to restore God's image. (See Chapter 2, pp. 27-31.)

Thus, hyssop oil, directed by our sincere intent to "create a clean heart and restore a right spirit within ourselves" can "blot out our transgressions" and erase the sinful tendencies (negative emotions) stored in cellular memory, thus releasing and cleansing the root cause of wrong action. (Psalm 51:9-10)

David's remorse was very intense and his repentance complete. The *Bible* contains no record that he ever committed such an act again. Repentance is an essential prelude to healing. (See Chapter 4, pp. 83-89.) In this Psalm we can learn much about the true meaning of repentance in the example set by David, the sinner who, in the end, accepted full responsibility for his actions and re-established his broken relationship with God.

Read John 19:29. Just before this verse Jesus realized that his trial on the cross was nearly accomplished. In order to fulfill the scripture, Psalm 69:21, "In my thirst they gave me vinegar to drink," he said to those standing by, "I thirst." Their response was to dip a sponge into some vinegar or sour wine and extend it to Jesus' mouth on a branch of hyssop. Why the use of hyssop is not clear. Neither is it clear why a branch of hyssop would even be present at a crucifixion site.

While the Roman soldiers were not known for their mercy, they did allow certain women of Jerusalem to bring narcotic-like mixtures to offer dying victims to ease their pain. Death by crucifixion is death by slow suffocation. As the victim gradually tires they can no longer lift themselves to breathe. As their lungs slowly fill up with fluid they die an agonizing death. The scent of hyssop has long been known for its ability to bring respiratory relief. In this case, perhaps hyssop was brought by the Jerusalem ladies of mercy as an aromatic to help the crucified breathe a little easier. Of course, when the sponge of sour wine on hyssop was offered to Jesus, he refused it, just as he refused the wine with myrrh offered just before he was nailed. In his role as the lamb slain for the sins of the world, his suffering for humankind was not to be mitigated by any man-given relief.

Another interpretation for the presence of hyssop at the crucifixion is this. When God established a convenant with the Hebrews in Egypt to deliver them from slavery, the night that he smote the firstborn sons of all the Egyptians he asked them to slaughter an unblemished lamb, dip a branch of hyssop in the blood, and strike the lintel and side posts of their doorways as a sign for the angel of death to pass over their dwellings sparing the sons of Israel. (Exodus 12) When God rescinded the covenant for Israel's long series of misdeeds in Jeremiah 3:8, he promised to make a new convenant to be "written in their hearts." (Jeremiah 31:31-34) During the Last Supper with Jesus and his disciples, Christ offers a new convenant in his blood. (Matthew 26:28; Mark 14:24; Luke 22:20) When the branch of hyssop was raised to Jesus on the cross, it was dipped in his blood as the lamb of God. (John 19:29) In this act, a new covenant was forged for all future generations, as described in Jeremiah 31, just as the covenant between God and the Hebrews had been affirmed in Egypt by a branch of hyssop dipped in the blood of the sacrificial lamb. In Egypt the the instructions were to strike the horizontal lintels and the vertical side posts with the hyssop branch. At Calvary the lintels and door posts were replaced by the vertical and horizontal beams of the cross. Thus, the symbology of God's promise in the Passover was repeated in the death of Jesus on the cross. That is an interpretation that I like, but you can decide for yourself about the meaning of the hyssop at Christ's crucifixion.

Mention that hyssop is in the mint family of plants which is the family of oils mostly used in the anointing technique called "raindrop technique." In raindrop we use oils of oregano, thyme, marjoram, basil, and peppermint, all of which are mints and all related to hyssop. Hyssop is a strong oil and can be irritating to some people's skin, but is safe in the palms and safe to inhale for everyone. It was sometimes diluted with carrier oil and rubbed on the chest for colds and bronchitis or inhaled as a decongestant and expectorant.

Tell a Personal Story

At this point I insert a personal experience with Biblical oils. If you have any personal stories, add them to your presentation in the appropriate places. Here is mine:

Healed of Pneumonia with Biblical Oils

Shortly after I published this book, my pastor came down with pneumonia. It was on a late Sunday evening. He was coughing up blood and had gone to the emergency room of a local hospital. He was given antibiotics, some cough medicine, and codeine as a narcotic to help him sleep. He returned home, took the medicines as prescribed, and only got worse.

His wife reported his declining condition to us at the start of choir practice on Wednesday night. According to her he was still coughing up blood, couldn't rest, couldn't eat, couldn't drink anything, and "hurt all over." She was becoming alarmed at his deteriorating condition and didn't know what to do. "He is just zonked out," she said, "and can hardly talk rationally or do anything for himself, and the codeine is tearing up his stomach, he has such a reaction. The doctors say they don't know how to stop the hemorrhaging in his lungs," she added shaking her head.

Normally, my wife and I keep a low profile in our church (United Methodist) so neither of us spoke up right away. 99% of the members of our church are totally wedded to allopathic medicine. Everyone in our church knows we do oils, but hardly anyone has been receptive to what we have to offer.

Suddenly, one of the choir members turned to the minister's wife saying, "You know, David and Lee Stewart have some oils that really helped my mother and maybe they can help the preacher." She then related that her mother had walking pneumonia the previous winter and for nearly three months had gone to doctors repeatedly, spending a great deal of money. She had taken many medicines and antibiotics and just kept getting worse. She said that she had mentioned using oils, but her mother wasn't interested.

"Finally, I had heard enough of my mother's complaining all the time," she said. "So I just went to her house one day and said, 'You know, mom, you've been taking the doctor's medicines for months now and you aren't getting any better. I want you quit taking all those drugs and we are going to try oils.' So I rubbed a blend of eucalyptus and melaleuca oils (R.C.™) on her chest and on her feet and put on a hot damp towel on her chest. I showed my dad, too, so he could do it several times a day and let her breathe the vapors. After two days she was cured of the pneumonia. So I know they work!" she stated emphatically.

I was watching the preacher's wife closely during this to see if there would be a response. There was none. So I figured she was not interested. At the end of choir practice, I quietly said to her, "I gave your husband a copy of my new book on healing oils about three weeks ago. I don't know if he has read it or if you have seen it." She replied that she had seen it, but had not read any of it. "You know, these oils really do work," I added. Then I shut up.

Choir was over at 8:00 PM. About 10:00 PM I got a phone call. It was the preacher's wife. "My husband wants you to bring over the oils," she said. "He's kind of drugged up right now, but how about tomorrow morning?" I said I would be there. I hung up and started praying silently for the preacher and asking for guidance as to what oils I should bring and how to use them.

Early the next morning, praying all the way, I went to the parsonage with a diffuser and four oils: Hyssop, Frankincense, Exodus II™, and R.C.™ Now I have to say, that I felt led by God on the first three oils, but since my faith was not perfect, I brought the R.C. along just for my own assurance, knowing that this blend had worked on pneumonia in other cases. But I also must add that as I was driving over I had no idea of what I was going to do with these oils except I had complete faith that God would guide me when I got there and would let me know whatever I needed to know at the time.

When I arrived, I found the preacher lying pale and listless in bed with his eyes only half open, almost in a stupor. "He's still coughing blood," said his wife.

Immediately I started the diffuser with a mixture of R.C. and Hyssop. I then helped her turn his body around on the bed so his head was as close to the diffuser as we could get it. I asked him to breathe deeply.

Dropping about eight to ten drops of Frankincense on his head, I rubbed it all over, explaining that I was anointing him with Frankincense like Moses anointed Aaron. He liked that and started pinking up right away.

I then put R.C. and Hyssop on the lung reflex areas of his feet, doing a special massage technique (vitaflex) across each foot several times. He liked that, too.

With his wife's help, I turned him over and raindropped Hyssop and R.C. on his upper back over the lungs and did some of the light stroking we do in raindrop. Then I turned him back on his back and raindropped R.C. and Hyssop on his chest, rubbing his chest all over. "I am anointing you in a manner similar to that done in ancient Biblical times," I explained to him and his wife. "Also," I added, "by dropping these oils a few inches above the skin, they are falling through your electromagnetic field and will start administering therapy to you before they even hit your body." The pastor and his wife both nodded in approval.

I then gave him the bottle of Exodus II and told him to tip it and put a drop or two in his mouth and swallow it. He did. I explained that these oils are mentioned in the book of Exodus and that Moses and Aaron used some of them to stop a plague recorded in the book of Numbers. "These oils will also help stop your pneumonia," I said.

He immediately responded exclaiming, "This is the best I have felt in days." About ten minutes later he began coughing up phlegm and clearing his lungs. ("The hyssop is working," I thought to myself.) "Look," he said excitedly, "there is no blood!" The hemorrhaging in his lungs had stopped.

I then left him with his wife peacefully resting with his head on a pillow next to the diffuser with instructions to breathe the vapors all day and take another drop or two of the Exodus blend from time to time. His wife had to go to work but told me that the house would be open if I wanted to come back later to check.

Returning that afternoon, I found him sitting up on his bed reading, *Healing Oils of the Bible*. "Pretty interesting book," he said. He was smiling and drinking some juice. "This is the first time I have been able to drink anything in a couple of days. I feel almost well."

I gave him another anointing of R.C. and Hyssop on his chest, rubbing it in well. He took another drop of Exodus orally. I anointed his head with Frankincense again, rubbing it thoroughly all over. He really liked that. I put some more Hyssop in his diffuser and then left him for the day.

The next morning about 10 A.M. I dropped in. He met me at the door with his shoes on, fully dressed. He had been working on his sermon and the church bulletin for the coming Sunday. "I didn't know a couple of days ago if I was going to be able to make it to church this week at all," he said with a big smile, "but thanks to your oils, I am just fine. I have a slight headache, but my breathing is clear. I don't think I have pneumonia any more. And you know," he added, "since you came with the oils yesterday, I haven't taken any of the doctor's prescriptions."

The next Sunday in church, he gave a testimony for his healing experience with the oils before the whole congregation and has been telling everyone about it ever since. He even conveyed his experience to the bishop and a number of his fellow ministers. A week later he came to my house to buy some books to give to friends saying, "If you ever want me to give a testimony on those oils, just tell me. I know that's what took care of my pneumonia."

Concluding Note: It is important to emphasize here that the initiative for receiving the oils and laying on of hands was from the minister and his wife, not me. If they would not have called and asked for the oils, I would not have gone nor pursued it any further. Their act of receptivity was essential for this healing to have taken place. (See Mark 6:10–11 and pages 80–83 of this book.)

END OF STORY

H. **MYRRH:** Comment that myrrh is the first oil to be mentioned in the *Bible* (Genesis 37:25) in the story of Joseph. (See Chapter 1.) When Joseph's jealous brothers wanted to kill him, a caravan of Midianites happened by, so they chose to sell him into slavery. The caravan was carrying " balm and myrrh." They were on their way to Egypt, where many years later, Joseph was elevated to an Egyptian ruler. At that time, when Joseph's brothers came to Egypt to procure food, they encountered Joseph as a king, not recognizing him as their brother. Among their gifts brought for the Egyptian Lord were "balm and myrrh." (Genesis 43:11)—the same two oils that had accompanied Joseph when he was carried into slavery.

Read Esther 2:12. (Esther's preparation as a bride for the King) Point out that not only was Esther massaged with oil of myrrh for six months in preparation for her marriage to the king, she was also anointed with many other oils (perfumes, ointments, or odors). Emotionally, myrrh has the effect of provoking a feeling of security and well being. Esther was an orphan, both of her parents having died. (Esther 2:7) Perhaps her six months of anointment with myrrh helped her to regain some of the sense of confidence and security she may have lost as a child.

Read Mark 15:23. (Offered to Jesus when he arrived at Golgotha to be crucified) Point out that not only is myrrh both the first oil to be mentioned in the *Bible* but also the last (Revelations 18:13). And not only is it in the first and last books of the *Bible*, it was one of the first and last oils to be received by Christ—first at his birth, and last at the cross where it was offered in the wine just before he was crucified.

Myrrh is, in fact, the most frequently mentioned oil of the *Bible*—156 times to be exact. (See Chapter Ten.)

When we read of the wise men in Matthew 2:11, myrrh was among the gifts offered. Mary would have particularly smiled at the gift of myrrh knowing that it was also meant for her and not just the babe. She would have known that she could rub it on her abdomen and remove the stretch marks from her pregnancy. She and Joseph would also have known that myrrh was to be rubbed on the umbilical cord of the newborn child to facilitate healing and prevent infection. She would probably have known, as a matter of folk wisdom, that the smell of myrrh on her body, as she breastfed the Christ child would promote a spiritual and emotional feeling of peace and security for both of them. By associating the smell of myrrh with the security of the mother's breast in infancy would establish an emotional memory that would resurrect these secure feelings any time there was the smell of myrrh throughout the rest of a person's life. The wise men would not have had to explain these things, because such understanding was common knowledge with the peoples of those times.

I.　**CALAMUS:**　Calamus oil is found in Exodus II, but is not available by itself.

J. **MYRTLE:**   **Read Esther 2:7** Explain that Esther's name in this passage is "Hadassah," which is Hebrew for Myrtle. During the year of preparation to become a bride for the king, myrtle, her namesake, was probably among the perfumes and odors applied. Mention that research by Daniel Penoel M.D. of France has found that oil of myrtle is effective for normalizing hormonal imbalances of the thyroid, hypothyroid, and ovaries, and soothing to the respiratory system.

K. **ONYCHA:**   Mentioned as an ingredient in holy incense in Exodus 30:34 (which was already read with Galbanum). Turn the open bottle of onycha upside down and comment that onycha is the heaviest of all the oils and won't even pour from the bottle. You need a toothpick to get some out. As you pass around the bottle with a toothpick, ask them if they note anything familiar about the smell. (It contains vanillin aldehyde, which gives it the smell of vanilla.) Note that oil of onycha is also mentioned in the *Talmud* as well as in the *Old Testament Apocrypha.* (See Appendix B.)

Onycha was valued for its ability to speed the healing of wounds and prevent infection. It has other names such as "Friar's Balm," "Benzoin," and "Java Frankincense." Its source was the Balsam or Benzoin Tree of the Far East from which a number of oils were imported into the Holy Land in ancient times including sandalwood and spikenard from India and Tibet.

L. **ROSE OF SHARON:** Comment that the rose of sharon of the *Bible* was *Cistus ladanifer,* also known as rock rose, cistus, ladanum, and labdanum, which is not the thorny bush with large multi-petaled flowers we know as a true rose. This beautiful rose has a soft honey-like scent, as well as an aromatic gum that exudes from the plant. Ancient shepherds noted that the gum of rock rose would become entangled in the wool of their sheep and goats and that when they had cuts or abrasions, they could rub this resin from the fur onto their wounds, and it would soothe and heal them. Research has been conducted on the cell regeneration properties of this oil.

Commercial Christian Anointing Oils

At this time you can bring out the vials of oil you may have procured from a Christian Book Store. The brand that I have been able to obtain in the Midwest is distributed by RODCO, Ltd., Lansing, Michigan (Their web page is www.rodco-ltd.com). Rodco oils may also be purchased from Cokesbury, a United Methodist pastoral supply company in Nashville, Tennessee, by visiting www.cokesbury.com or by calling (800) 672-1789. They have two oils sold in small clear 1/4 oz. glass vials for around $4-5 each. One of these Rodco oils is said to be "Scented Anointing Oil of Healing Blessing" containing frankincense and myrrh. The other is labeled as "Rose of Sharon Anointing Oil." Now that your audience has smelled real frankincense, real myrrh, and real rose of sharon, pass these around to see if they can detect the presence of any of these real oils.

The first thing I point out as being suspect is that the containers are clear transparent glass, which is not appropriate for any essential oil. Light causes essential oils to polymerize. Polymerization is where small molecules link together forming chains and growing into large molecules. The healing power of essential oils is because of their tiny molecules that can penetrate tissues and cell walls and administer therapy to our bodies at those levels. When molecules are too big, they cannot heal.

Thus, essential oils must be protected from light. Furthermore, the small molecular structure is what makes it possible to smell essential oils. When their molecules grow too large by polymerization, their fragrance vanishes as well. So clear glass bottles is the first clue that these oils may not be what they say they are.

I always read the label to the audience which says: "This product is genuine." Now that is a non-statement if ever I heard one. It doesn't say genuine "what." That statement applies to everything. Everything is genuine something, even the soil on your shoes. The label goes on to say, "All imported ingredients," which is, again, a non-statement, telling us nothing. Then we read "Frankincense and myrrh is (sic) blended with pure golden juice pressed from choice hand-picked fruit of the olive tree." I then pass the bottle around for the audience to sniff to see if they can detect any frankincense or myrrh.

I then comment on the olive oil. The *Bible* clearly states that the only grade of olive oil suitable as a carrier for essential oils for anointing purposes is "first oil" or "beaten oil." (Exodus 27:20; 29:40; Leviticus 24:2; Numbers 28:5) (Also see Chapter Eleven of this book.) Today first oil is called "virgin oil." Virgin olive oil has a fragrance and flavor and is not pressed from the fruit, but drained from the crushed fruit. Pressed oil (which is mentioned on the label of the Christian book store oil) is actually the Biblical "second" oil and was not acceptable as an offering to the temple. Pressed oil has no flavor and no fragrance. It is squeezed from the olives after the virgin or first oil has been extracted. In other words, these commercial anointing oils don't even use the right grade of olive, which anyone can ascertain by smelling it. They used the cheapest odorless olive oil they could find. The whole product is a fraud.

Now check the other commercial brand labeled as "Rose of Sharon." Here, again, the label says "This product is genuine." It also says "blended to perfection with the highest quality ingredients procurable," another meaningless statement. "It's scent is lovely," says the label, "one of the world's most incredible fragrances." Nowhere does it say that actual oil of rose of sharon is an ingredient. Again, I ask my audience to be the experts and tell me if this is, indeed, the rose of sharon and if the olive carrier is first oil, as the *Bible* would have it, or second.

As your audience will recognize, the fragrance of that brand is probably some synthetic rose fragrance and certainly not real rock rose or rose of sharon. And again, there is no fragrance to the oil carrier, identifying it as cheap second grade. Thus another fraud is uncovered.

Look for AFNOR

I then take the opportunity to warn them about the quality of essential oils in general, saying that you can't just go to the nearest health food store or herb shop and buy whatever oils are on the shelf and expect them to be therapeutic grade like the healing oils of the *Bible*. If you don't get therapeutic grade oils, then you won't get the healing results either. Look for the designation "AFNOR" on the label. Only then do you have confirmation that the oil is genuinely therapeutic grade.

M. **SPIKENARD:** Point out that Spikenard was one of the last oils received by Jesus before his arrest in Jerusalem. Ask if they remember the woman coming to one of Jesus' last meals and anointing him with a precious ointment? Then ask the group whether Jesus was anointed on his head or on his feet and who was the woman? Get a poll of opinions? Then Read the following scriptures in the order given: Read **Matthew 26:6-7, Luke 7:36-38, Mark 14:3, John 12:1-3**. The four versions seem contradictory and pose a series of questions: Who was the woman? Where did the incident take place? When did it take place? What was contained in the ointment applied? Was it applied to Jesus' head or to his feet?

Tell them that this is the "Mystery of the Anointing Woman" which is completely solved in Chapter Ten of the book *Healing Oils of the Bible.* For purposes of this program you can say that the oil was not just spikenard, it was a blend of both spikenard and myrrh. You can also say that the oil was applied to both Jesus' head and to his feet because there were actually three incidents of anointing. One two days before the passover in the house of Simon the Leper where the anointment was on his head, another in the house of Lazarus six days before the passover where the oil was poured over his feet, and yet third anointment early in Jesus' ministry.

The amount of oil used was about one litra which would be worth almost $2000 in today's currency. This was equivalent to a year's wages for a common laborer at that time and place.

The application of both spikenard and myrrh in the last week of Jesus life has some interesting implications. Both of these oils are known for their ability to heal wounds and scar tissue. In John 12:3-7, where Jesus is anointed by Mary, the sister of Lazarus, six days before his death, Judas objects to such a valuable commodity being used to anoint Jesus feet when it could have been sold for a substantial amount and distributed to the poor. Jesus' response to Judas was to say,

"Leave her alone. She bought it for the day of my burial."

Myrrh was a customary burial oil, but spikenard was not. We read in Isaiah 53:5, "He was wounded for our transgressions, he was bruised for our iniquities...and with his stripes we are healed." Jesus knew of he was to receive a brutal flogging from the Roman soldiers in less than a week, just prior to his death. He knew his body would be covered with deep cuts and bruises in addition to the penetrating wounds of the cross. He also knew a miracle was to take place during his burial. Except for the scars on his feet, hands, and side, his injuries would all be healed without a trace.

While Jesus' healing and resurrection was act of God, and not the result of any oils applied just before or after his death, it is interesting that the oils Jesus received, twice in the last week of his life, are precisely the ointments that would have been chosen to treat such wounds to effect healing with little or no scar tissue. Jesus' comment to Judas was was as if he was affirming the appropriateness of these essential oils from which his body could well benefit during his ordeal—before, during, and after the cross—as well as in the tomb, during his burial, when his healing took place.

CONCLUDING REMARKS

The leader should **Read Mark 6:7, 10-13,** and make the following concluding comments. There are four major points to be made:

(1) Mark 10-11 gives Jesus' advice on what to do when we find relatives or friends who are sick and could benefit from essential oils but who are unreceptive and, perhaps critical of what we may offer them out of concern and in good faith. Jesus says forget them and move on. Don't waste your time. Find people who are receptive and ready and administer to them. The same advice is given in Luke 10:1-12. (See Chapter Four, section on "Anointing to Heal as Taught by Christ.")

(2) Mark 6:12 tells us that healing has to be accompanied with repentance. (See Chapter Four, section entitled "The Cause of Sickness.")

(3) Mark 6:13 (first part) mentions casting out devils. This is another point to be made. (See Chapter Four, section entitled "Casting out Devils.")

(4) Mark 6:13 (last part) says that the disciples anointed with oil many that were sick and healed them. (See Chapter Four, section entitled "Anointing With Oils.")

In conclusion, say words to the effect: "Those of us who work with these oils and teach others how to use them and who practice raindrop technique and other methods of anointing feel that we are carrying on the work of Christ as taught to his disciples and as expressed in this passage of Mark." If you have time, conclude by reading **James 5:14** and immediately follow the reading of that passage with words such as these: "It is our hope that the art and practice of healing will be returned to the church, as expressed in James, and as it was practiced by Christ's disciples and the early Christian Church. This is the end of our program. Thank you for coming."

Final Announcements and Prayer

Before people leave, you may want to announce any scheduled future programs if you haven't already done that in the beginning.

You can announce that if people want more in-depth information on using the oils, you have copies of the EODR for sale, and if they want more complete information on the *Healing Oils of the Bible*, you may have some copies of that book for sale, also. Or if you wish, you can give them order blanks as to where they can obtain both books.

This is also where you would announce that you have information on how to obtain therapeutic grade oils and, perhaps, have some free tapes and literature for those who wish. Invite them to stay and talk or ask questions if they want to. If the program has been held in a church, you will want to close with prayer, which is a good idea anywhere you do this program.

NOTE: There is a 2-hour video called "Healing Oils of the *Bible*." of Dr. Stewart doing the *Bible* Oils program available from CARE (Ordering info on page 325). A perfect teaching tool for you to learn how to do the program yourself. Can also be shown as a program, in and of itself, while passing around the oils.

Appendix A
Catalogue of Bible Citations for Essential Oils & Aromatic Plants

This appendix is the documentation for Chapter Five, entitled "How Many Oils are Mentioned in the *Bible*?" That chapter gives the rationale of how and why the *Bible* passages of this compilation were chosen so that you can understand the thinking and either agree or disagree with the totals that have been tabulated.

In a number of cases, the *Bible* mentions aromatic plants such as Anise, Bay, Coriander, Cumin, Cypress, Dill, Fir, Henna (Camphire), Juniper, Mint, Mustard, Myrtle, Pine, Rose, Rue, Shittim (Acacia), Terebinth, and Wormwood without specifically stating that essential oils were extracted from them. In some cases, the aromatic wood was also used for lumber. That these were, in fact, sources of oils in Biblical times can be found in references outside of the *Bible*. See Appendix C for more on this.

According to our research, there are 33 species of aromatic plants given in the *Bible* from which essential oils were produced. Depending on the way you count them, there are as many as 1035 references to essential oils and/or the plants that produced them in the *Old Testament and New Testament*. 642 citations are given in this Appendix, many of which refer to more than one oil, which is how we get 1035 references from 642 citations.

There are another 68 mentions of oils and aromatic plants, including three additional species, in the *Old Testament Apocrypha* (See Appendix B).

This Appendix contains five tables as follows:

TABLE ONE-A
Essential Oils and/or Aromatic Plants
of the *Bible* (33 species)

TABLE TWO-A
Specific Biblical References to Essential Oils
and/or Aromatic Plants (262 citations)

TABLE THREE-A
Indirect Biblical References to Essential Oils
and/or Aromatic Plants (140 citations)

TABLE FOUR-A
General Biblical References to Essential Oils
and/or Aromatic Plants (240 citations)

TABLE FIVE-A
Books of the *Bible* that Mention Essential Oils
and/or Aromatic Plants (42 Books)

The references to oils and plants in this Appendix are
of are of three types:

1. Specific References: An essential oil or oil bearing plant is referred to by name as a unique species that
has been identified by modern botanical nomenclature.
There are 33 species mentioned a total of 262 times this
way. (See Tables One-A and Four-A.)

2.   Indirect References: An essential oil or oils
referred to indirectly without mention of specific names,
but where the names can be identified. This includes
phrases such as "holy anointing oil" or "holy incense"
where the specific oil ingredients are known, but not
given at that point in the Biblical text. There are 140
such references. (See Table Two-A.)

3. General References: An essential oil or oils is definitely implied, but the exact species are not determinable. This includes mentions of such things as ointments, perfumes, and spices, where the use of aromatic plant oils is certain, but the names of the species are not known. There are 240 such references. (See Table Three-A.)

A Request for Your Assistance

The following tabulations of Biblical references to essential oils and/or their plant sources is intended to be exhaustive. However, as would be the case for any project of this magnitude, there are probably some errors and omissions.

If you find any additional references we have missed or items to be corrected, we would appreciate that information to add to future editions of this catalogue.

Format for Table One-A

We begin with Table One-A on the next page, which is a list of the thirty-three specifically referenced species of oils and/or oil-producing plants of the *Bible*. The information in Table One is formatted as follows:

• **First: The English Biblical name and the number of explicit Biblical mentions is given in bold type along with the pronunciation where the strong syllable is underlined.**

• Second: When other common names in English exist they are given in parentheses in regular type.

• Third: The Hebrew and/or Greek or Latin names are given in regular type with their meanings where obtainable.

• *Fourth: The scientific names are given in italics with their meanings from the Latin where known.*

TABLE ONE-A

Essential Oils and/or Aromatic Plants
Of the Bible
(33 Species)
(See Table Four-A for the Scriptural Citations)

1. ALOES 5x   **(a̱ . loes)**
(Sandalwood, Trees of Lign, Lign-aloes)
Heb. ahaloth or ahalim. Grk. aloes, meaning "noble."
Santalum album (S.= sanskrit name of the tree;
    a.= white bark)

2. ANISE 1x   **(a̱ . nise)**
Grk. anethon, which can also mean dill or cumin
Pimpenella anisum (P.= as if composed of pepper-
    corns; a.= anise)

3. BALM 6x
(Balsam, Balm of Gilead, Balm of Mecca,
    Balm of Jericho)
Heb. tsori or tseri, meaning "medicine gum"
Commiphora opobalsamum (C.= gum bearing;
    o.= juice from the balm tree)

4. BAY 1x
(Bay Laurel)
Heb. esrach, meaning "native born"
Laurilus nobilis (L.=evergreens; n.=notable or noble}

5. BDELLIUM 1x   **(bde̱l . li. um)**
Heb. bedolach, meaning "bitter oily gum"
Commiphora africana (C.= gum bearing; a.= from
    Africa.)

6. CALAMUS 3x   (<u>cal</u> . a. mus)
(Aromatic Cane)
Heb. qaneh, meaning "a reed or cane."
   Grk. kalamos, meaning "stalk, stem or reed"
Acorus calamus (A.= sweet flag; c.= reedlike)

7. CASSIA 3x   (<u>cas</u> . si. a)
(Oriental Cinnamon)
Heb. qiddah, meaning "amber," or qetsioth, meaning
   "bark like cinnamon" Grk. kasia = acacia
Cinnamomum cassia (C.= like cinnamon; c.=
   Greek name for trees resembling acacias)

8. CEDARWOOD 70x   (<u>cee</u> . dar. wood)
(Juniper)
Heb. erez, meaning "hard wood" Gr. kedros, mean-
   ing "resinous tree"
Cedrus libani/atlantica (C.= true cedar; l.= of Lebanon;
   a.= of the Atlas Mountains of Greece)

9. CINNAMON 4x   (<u>sin</u> . na. mon)
Heb. qinnamon. Grk. kinamomon
Cinnamomum verum (C.= cinnamon; v.= true)

10. CORIANDER 2x   (co. ree. <u>an</u> . der)
Heb. gad, meaning "round aromatic seed"
   Grk. koriannon, after koris, a bug that smells
   like the leaves of the plant.
Coriandrum sativum (C.= ancient name for the
   plant; s.= that which is sown or grown

11. CUMIN 4x   (<u>coo</u> . men)
(Cumin, Cumino)
Heb. kammon, meaning "sharp smell." Grk. kumi-
   non, "the cumin plant"
Cuminum cyminum (C.= aromatic herb; c.= cumin
   seed)

TABLE ONE-A . . . Oils & Aromatics cont'd

---

12. CYPRESS 5x   (<u>sy</u> . press)
(Gopherwood, Oil Tree)
Heb. tirzah. Grk. kyparissos
Cupressus sempervirens (C.= cypress tree;
    s.= everlasting or always green)

13. DILL 3x
(Fitches, Nutmeg Flower)
Heb. ketsach, which can also mean black cumin
Anethum graveolens (A.= dill or anise; g.= heavily
    scented)

14. FIR 21x
(Silver Fir)
Heb. berosh or bero him, both of which can also
    mean pine or cypress
Abies alba (A.= ancient name for fir trees; a.=
    white bark)

15. FRANKINCENSE 22x   (<u>frank</u> . in. cents)
(Incense, Olibanum)
Heb. lebonah. Grk. olibanos. Old Lat. olibanum. All
    derived from the Arabic. al luban, meaning "milk."
    In Late Latin, the language used in the Vulgate
    or original Catholic Bible, it became francum incen-
    sum, meaning literally, "real, pure, or true incense,"
    which is where the King James Bible translators
    got the English expression "Frankincense" we use
    today.
Boswellia carteri (B.= after Scottish botanist Dr.
    John Boswell; c.= after British surgeon and
    herbologist Dr. H.J. Carter who first identified
    the species and brought samples to England.

16. GALBANUM 1x   (**gal** . ba. num)
(Galban)
Heb. chelbanah or khelbnah, meaning "fatness"
Ferula Gummosa (F.= the giant fennel, a rod or a
   walking stick; g.= gummy resin)

17. HENNA 2x   (**hen** . na
(Camphire, Privet)
   Heb. kopher, meaning "reddish brown" after a
   dye used for coloring fingers, nails, and hair in
   Biblical times. The white flowers were aromatic.
Lawsonia inermis (L.=after Scottish botanist Dr.
   John Lawson; i.= unarmed or having no thorns)

18. HYSSOP 12x   (**hiss** . up)
(Organy)
Heb. ezob. Grk. hussopos. both meaning
   "aromatic plant"
Hyssopus officinalis (H.= aromatic plant;
   o.= officially used in medicine

19. JUNIPER 4x   (**jew** . ni. per)
(Broom Tree, Cedar)
Heb. rothem, meaning "broom," because the
   Israelites used juniper boughs as brooms to
   sweep their floors and campgrounds.
Juniperus osteosperma (J.= juniper; o.= bone
   seed)

20. MINT 2x
(Horse Mint)
Grk. heduosmon
Mentha Longifolia (M.= mint; l.= long-leafed)

TABLE ONE-A . . . Oils & Aromatics cont'd

---

21. MUSTARD SEED 5x
Grk. sinapi
Brassica nigra (B.= cabbage; n.= black)

22. MYRRH 18x   (murr)
(Balm, Balsam, Bdellium, Ladanum, Stacte)
Heb. mor. Grk. smurna, smurnizo, or muron. All of
   which mean "bitter" in both languages
Commiphora myrrha (C.= gum bearing; m.= bitter)

23. MYRTLE 6x   (mur . tul)
Heb. hadas. The feminine form of the word is
   Hadassah, which was Esther's other name
   as given in Esther 2:7
Myrtus communis (M.= myrtle; c.= common)

24. ONYCHA 1x   (on . i. keh)
(Benzoin, Friar's Balm, Frankincense of Java)
Heb. shechelet, from an Arabic word referring to
   the "husks of wheat or barley"
Styrax benzoin (S.= fragrant gum; b.= incense
   of Java)

25. PINE 2x
(Oil Tree)
Heb. tidhar, which can also mean elm or fir tree.
   Also called "ets shemen" in Hebrew, meaning
   "a tree of oil, very fruitful"
Pinus sylvestris (P.= pine tree; s.= of the forest)

26. ROSE OF ISAIAH 1x   **(ai. <u>zay</u> . ah)**
(Meadow Saffron, Crocus, Narcissus)
Heb. chabatstsele (colorful flower)
Narcissus tazetta (N.= narcotic, numbness, stupor;
    t.= like a little cup or vase)

27. ROSE OF SHARON 1x   **(sha. <u>rone</u>)**
(Cistus, Ladanum, Labdanum, Rock Rose)
Heb. chabatstsele (colorful flower)
Cistus ladanifer (C.= rock rose; l. = from the Greek
    ledon and Arabic ladon referring to a dark resin
    used as chewing gum in ancient times)

28. RUE 1x   **(roo)**
Grk. peganon
Ruta graveolens (R.= rue; g.= heavily scented)

29. SAFFRON 1x   **(<u>saf</u> . fron)**
(Indian Saffron, Crocus)
Heb. karkom
Crocus sativus (C.= orange-yellow; s.= that which
    is sown or grown)

30. SHITTAH 26x   **(<u>sheet</u> . ah)**
(Acacia, Arabic Gum Tree, Egyptian Thorn)
(Shittim is the plural form of shittah)
Heb. Shittah. Grk. akakia = "sharp pointed"
Acacia arabica (A.= thorn or point; a.= from
Arabia)

TABLE ONE-A . . . Oils & Aromatics cont'd

STACTE   (<u>stack</u> . tee)   **(see myrrh)**

31. SPIKENARD 7x   (<u>spike</u> . nard)
(Nard)
Heb. nerd. Grk. nardos pistikos = "genuine nard"
Nardostachys jatamansi (N.= from a Persian word
referring to the nard plant; j.= the Sanskrit name
of the plant from where it is found in India.

32. TEREBINTH 13x   (<u>ter</u>. a. binth)
(Turpentine Tree, Palestinian Oak, Pistachio)
Heb. elah or allah
Pistacia terebinthus var. palestina (P.= pistachio
tree; t.= turpentine tree; p.=from Palestine

33. WORMWOOD 8x
Heb. laana. Grk. absinthos = bitter, undrinkable
Artemesia judiaca var. absinthia (A.= Artemis,
Greek moon goddess; j.= the land of Judah;
a.= bitter)

NOTE: In the tables that follow, where a reference word appears twice in the same verse, they are cited as "a" and "b" as is seen in Leviticus 16:13a, 13b on the next page. Such instances are counted as two Biblical mentions.

TABLE TWO-A

Specific Biblical References to
Essential Oils and/or Aromatic Plants
(There are 261 Citations & 33 Species in this Table)
(Also see Table One-A)

ACACIA (See Shittim)

ALOES (SANDALWOOD) (Santalum album)   5x
Numbers 24:6
Psalms 45:8
Proverbs 7:17
Song of Solomon 4:14
John 19:39

ANISE (Pimpenella anisum)   1x
Matthew 23:23

BALM (Commiphora opobalsamum)   6x
Genesis 37:25; 43:11
Jeremiah 8:22; 46:22; 51:8
Ezekiel 27:17

BAY (Laurilus nobilis)   1x
Psalms 37:35

BDELLIUM (Commiphora africana)   1x
Numbers 11:7

CALAMUS (Acorus calamus)   3x
Exodus 30:23
Song of Solomon 4:14
Ezekiel 27:19

| **TABLE TWO-A . . . Biblical Citations cont'd** |

CEDARWOOD as oil (Cedrus libani)   5x

Leviticus 14:4, 6, 49, 52
Numbers 19:6

CEDARWOOD as aromatic lumber(C. libani)   25x

II Samuel 7:2, 7
I Kings 5:8; 6:9, 10, 15, 16, 18, 20, 36; 7:2, 3, 7, 12
I Chronicles 14:1; 17:1, 6; 22:4
II Chronicles 2:3
Song of Solomon 1:17; 8:9
Jeremiah 22:14, 15
Ezekiel 27:24
Zephaniah 2:14

CEDARS as living aromatic trees (C. libani)   40x

Numbers 24:6
Judges 9:15
II Samuel 5:11
I Kings 4:33; 5:6, 10; 7:11; 9:11; 10:27
II Kings 14:9; 19:23
I Chronicles 22:4
II Chronicles 1:15; 2:8; 9:27; 25:18
Ezra 3:7
Job 40:17
Psalms 29:5; 80:20; 92:12; 104:16; 148:9
Song of Solomon 5:15
Isaiah 2:15; 9:20; 14:8; 37:24; 41:19; 44:14
Jeremiah 22:7
Ezekiel 17:3, 22, 23; 27:5; 31:3, 8
Amos 2:9
Zechariah 11:1, 2

CASSIA (Cinnamomum Cassia) 3x
Exodus 30:24
Ezekiel 27:19
Psalm 45:8

CINNAMON (Cinnamomum verum) 4x
Exodus 30:23
Proverbs 7:17
Song of Solomon 4:14
Revelation 18:3

CORIANDER (Coriandrum sativum) 2x
Exodus 16:31
Numbers 11:7

CUMIN (Cuminum cyminum) 4x
isaiah 28:25, 27a, 27b
Matthew 23:23

CYPRESS (Cupressus sempervirens) 5x
Genesis 6:14
Isaiah 41:19; 44:14
I Kings 9:11
Song of Solomon 1:17

DILL (Anethum graveolens) 3x
Isaiah 28:25, 27
Matthew 23:23

TABLE TWO-A . . . Biblical Citations cont'd

FIR as an aromatic lumber(Abies alba)   8x
II Samuel 6:5
I Kings 5:8, 10; 6:15, 34; 9:11
II Chronicles 3:5
Song of Solomon 1:17

FIR as living aromatic trees(Abies alba)   13x
II Kings 19:23
II Chronicles 2:8
Psalms 104:17
Isaiah 14:8; 37:24; 41:19; 55:13; 60:13
Ezekiel 27:5; 31:8
Hosea 14:8
Nahum 2:3
Zechariah 11:2

FRANKINCENSE (Boswellia carteri)   22x
Exodus 30:34
Leviticus 2:1, 15, 16; 5:11; 6:15; 24:7
Numbers 5:15
I Chronicles 9:29
Nehemiah 13:5, 9
Song of Solomon 3:6; 4:6, 14
Isaiah 43:23; 60:6; 66:3
Jeremiah 6:20; 17:26; 41:5
Matthew 2:11
Revelation 18:13

GALBANUM (Ferula gummosa)   1x
Exodus 30:34

HENNA (CAMPHIRE) (Lawsonia inermis) 2x
Song of Solomon 1:14; 4:13

HYSSOP (Hyssopus officinalis) 12x
Exodus 12:22
Leviticus 14:4, 6, 49, 51, 52
Numbers 19:6, 18
I Kings 4:33
Psalms 51:7
John 19:29
Hebrews 9:19

JUNIPER (Juniperus osteosperma) 4x
I Kings 19:4, 5
Job 30:4
Psalms 120:4

MINT (HORSE MINT) (Mentha longifolia) 2x
Matthew 23:23
Luke 11:42

MUSTARD SEED (Brassica nigra) 5x
Matthew 13:31; 17:20
Mark 4:31
Luke 13:19; 17:6

MYRRH (Commiphora myrrha) 18x
Genesis 37:25; 43:11
Exodus 30:23, 34
Esther 2:12
Psalms 45:8
Proverbs 7:17
Song of Solomon 1:13; 3:6; 4:6, 14; 5:1, 5a, 5b, 13
Matthew 2:11
Mark 15:23
John 19:39

TABLE TWO-A . . . Biblical Citations cont'd

MYRTLE (Myrtus communis)   6x
Nehemiah 8:15
Isaiah 41:19; 55:13
Zechariah 1:8, 10, 11

ONYCHA (Styrax benzoin)   1x
Exodus 30:34

PINE (Pinus sylvestris)   2x
Nehemiah 8:15
Isaiah 41:19; 60:13

ROSE OF ISAIAH (Narcissus tazetta)   1x
Isaiah 35:1

ROSE OF SHARON (Cistus ladanifer)   1x
Song of Solomon 2:1

RUE (Ruta graveolens)   1x
Luke 11:42

SAFFRON (Crocus sativus)   1x
Song of Solomon 4:14

SANDALWOOD (See Aloes)   5x

SHITTAH (ACACIA) (Acacia arabica)   26x
Exodus 25:5. 10, 13, 23, 28; 26:15, 26, 32, 37;
27:1, 6; 30:1, 5; 35:7, 24; 36:20, 31, 36; 37:1, 4,
10, 25; 38:1, 6
Deuteronomy 10:3
Isaiah 41:19

SPIKENARD (Nardostachys jatamansi)   7x
Song of Solomon 1:2; 4:13, 14
Matthew 26:7
Mark 14:3
Luke 7:37
John 12:3

TEREBINTH (Pistacia terebinthus)   13x
Genesis 35:4
Judges 6:11, 19
Joshua 24:26
II Samuel 18:9a, 9b, 10, 14
I Kings 13:14
I Chronicles 10:12
Isaiah 1:30; 6:13
Ezekiel 6:13

WORMWOOD (Artemisia judiaca)   8x
Deuteronomy 29:18
Proverbs 5:4
Jeremiah 9:15; 23:15
Lamentations 3:15, 19
Revelations 8:11a, 11b

NOTE: There are 261 specific references and 33 species in this table. For 138 additional Biblical mentions of Calamus, Cassia, Cedarwood, Cinnamon, Frankincense, Galbanum, Myrrh, Onycha, and Spikenard, see Table Three-A of this Appendix entitled "Indirect Biblical References to Essential Oils..."

TABLE THREE-A

Indirect Biblical References
To Essential Oils and/or Aromatic Plants

Indirect references are those where specific oils are not named but the use of essential oils and their species are implied and identifiable. There are 146 such references. 140 are in this Table, the other six are where "lebonah" (Heb. for frankincense) was translated as "incense." These six citations are given under frankincense in Table Two-A.

HOLY INCENSE 54x
Myrrh, Onycha, Galbanum, Frankincense
(defined in Exodus 30:34-37)

Exodus 25:6; 30:1, 7, 8, 27; 31:8; 35:8, 15, 28;
      37:25, 29; 39:38; 40:5, 27
Leviticus 16:12, 13a, 13b
Numbers 4:16; 7:14, 20, 26, 32, 38, 44, 50, 56, 62, 68,
75, 80, 86; 16:7, 17, 18, 35, 40, 46, 47
Deuteronomy 33:10
I Samuel 2:28
I Chronicles 6:49; 28:18
II Chronicles 2:4; 13:11; 26:16; 29:7
Ezekiel 8:11; 16:18; 23:41
Luke 1:9, 10, 11
Revelation 8:3, 4

EMBALMING 4x
Myrrh, Frankincense, Cedarwood,
(In that time and place these three oils
were always used for embalming)
Genesis 50:2a, 2b, 3, 20

HOLY ANOINTING OIL 65x
Myrrh, Cinnamon, Calamus, Cassia
(defined in Exodus 30: 22-25)

Exodus 25:6; 28:47; 29:2, 7, 21, 36; 30:25, 26, 30, 31;
      31:11; 35:8, 15, 28; 37:29; 39:38;
      40:9, 10, 11, 13, 15
Leviticus 2:4; 4:3, 5, 16; 6:22; 7:12, 35a, 35b, 36;
      8:2, 10, 11, 12, 30; 10:7; 16:32; 21:10, 12
Numbers 3:3; 4:6; 7:1, 10, 84, 88; 18:8; 35:25
I Samuel 2:35; 10:1; 16:1, 13
II Samuel 1:21
I Kings 1:39; 19:16
II Kings 9:1, 3, 6
Psalms 89:20; 92:10
Isaiah 10:27; 21:5; 61:6
Ezekiel 16:9
Daniel 9:24

OINTMENT 14x
Myrrh, Spikenard
(In the Greek, the N.T. references to "ointment" all refer to
spikenard blended with myrrh)

Matthew 26:7, 9, 12
Mark 14:3, 4
Luke 7:37, 38, 46; 23:56
John 11:2; 12:3a, 3b, 5
Revelation 18:13

SPICES 1x
Myrrh, Onycha, Galbanum, Frankincense,
Cinnamon, Calamus, Cassia
(The word "spices" in this verse refers specifically to the
ingredients in holy incense and anointing oil)

Exodus 25:6

TABLE FOUR-A

General Biblical References
To Essential Oils and/or Aromatic Plants

General References are those where a reference to essential oils is sure, but the specific oils are not named and cannot be identified. There are 240 such mentions. This class of citations includes the following eleven categories: Sweet Savors 50x, Spices 36x, Anointing Kings 61x, Anointing People 27x, Censers 20x, Ointment 17x, Incense (but not "holy incense") 8x, Odors 7x, Perfume 6x, Oils of Joy 4x, Context 4x.

SWEET SAVORS 50x

Genesis 8:21
Exodus 5:21; 29:18, 25
Leviticus 1:9, 13, 17; 2:2, 9, 12; 3:5, 16; 4:31; 6:15, 21;
        8:21, 28; 17:6; 23:13, 18; 26:31
Numbers 15:3, 7, 10, 13, 14, 24; 18:17; 28:2, 6, 8, 13,
        24, 27; 29:2, 6, 8, 13, 36
Ezra 6:10
Song of Solomon 1:3
Ezekiel 6:13; 16:19; 20:28, 41
Ephesians 5:2
II Corinthians 2:14, 15, 16a, 16b

ODORS 7x

Leviticus 26:31
Esther 2:12
Daniel 2:46
John 12:3
Philippians 4:18
Revelation 5:8; 18:13

SPICES 36x
Genesis 37:25; 43:11
Exodus 30:23, 34a, 34b; 35:8, 28; 37:29
I Kings 10:2, 10a, 10b, 15, 25
II Kings 20:13
I Chronicles 9:29, 30
II Chronicles 9:1, 9a, 9b, 24; 32:27
Song of Solomon 4:10, 14, 16; 5:1, 13; 6:2; 8:2, 14
Isaiah 39:2
Ezekiel 24:10; 27:22
Mark 16:1
Luke 23:56; 24:1
John 19:40

KINGS ANOINTED WITH OIL 61x
(Kings were always anointed with oils containing fragrances
and sometimes even with the holy anointing oil of Exodus
30:22-25)
Judges 9:8, 15
I Samuel 2:10; 9:16; 10:1; 12:3, 5; 15:1, 17; 16:3, 12, 13;
      24:6a, 6b, 10; 26:9, 11, 16, 23
II Samuel 1:14, 16; 2:4, 7; 3:39; 5:3, 17; 12:7; 19:10, 21;
      22:51; 23:1
I Kings 1:34, 39, 45; 5:1; 19:15, 16
II Kings 9:3, 6, 12; 11:2; 23:30
I Chronicles 11:3; 14:8; 16:22; 29:22
II Chronicles 6:42; 22:7; 23:11
Psalms 18:50; 20:6; 23:5; 28:8; 84:9; 89:38, 51; 92:10;
105:15; 132:10. 17
Isaiah 45:1

TABLE FOUR-A . . . General References cont'd

PEOPLE ANOINTED WITH OIL 27x
(Oil containing aromatics, but not necessarily "holy anointing oil." See Table Two-A for holy anointing oil.)

Exodus 29:2, 21
Leviticus 2:4; 8:10, 12; 21:10
Numbers 35:25
Deuteronomy 28:40
Ruth 3:3
I Samuel 10:1
II Samuel 12:20; 14:2
I Kings 9:3
II Kings 9:6
Ii Chronicles 28:15
Psalms 45:7; 92:10

Ezekiel 16:9
Daniel 10:3
Amos 6:6
Micah 6:15
Matthew 6:17
Mark 6:13; 16:1
Luke 7:38, 40, 46; 10:34
John 4:2; 12:3
Hebrews 1:9
James 5:14
Revelations 3:18

INCENSE BURNING CENSERS 20x
Leviticus 10:1; 16:12
Numbers 4:14; 16:6, 17a, 17b, 17c, 18, 37, 38, 39, 46
I Kings 7:50
II Chronicles 4:22; 26:19
Ezekiel 8:11
Hebrews 9:4
Revelations 8:3, 5

ESSENTIAL OILS IMPLIED BY CONTEXT 4x
Deuteronomy 7:13
I Kings 5:11
Proverbs 21:20
Hosea 12:1

OINTMENT 17x

Exodus 30:25
II Kings 20:13
I Chronicles 9:30
Job 41:31
Psalms 133:2
Proverbs 27:9, 16
Ecclesiastes 7:1; 9:8; 10:1
Song of Solomon 1:3a, 3b; 4:10
Isaiah 1:6; 39:2; 57:9
Amos 6:6

INCENSE 8x

(But not "holy incense." See Table Two-A for that)
Exodus 30:9
Leviticus 10:1
II Chronicles 30:14
Isaiah 1:13
Psalms 66:15; 141:2
Jeremiah 44:21
Malachi 1:11

PERFUME 6x

Exodus 30:35, 37
Proverbs 7:17; 27:9
Song of Solomon 3:6
Isaiah 57:9

OILS OF JOY and GLADNESS 4x

Psalms 45:7
Proverbs 22:9
Isaiah 61:3
Hebrews 1:9

TABLE FIVE-A

Books of the Bible that Mention Essential Oils and/or Aromatic Plants

Most of the books of the Bible mention oils and aromatic plants: 36 out of 39 of the books of the Old Testament (92%) and 10 out of 27 of the books of the New Testament (37%). In total, 46 out of 66 (70%) or over two-thirds of the books of the Bible have some mention of essential oils and/or the aromatic plants from which they are derived.The following tabulation indicates what specific books contain by use of the following key:

1 = Aloes or Sandalwood	23 = Myrtle
2 = Anise	24 = Onycha
3 = Balm	25 = Pine
4 = Bay	26 = Rose of Isaiah
5 = Bdellium	27 = Rose of Sharon
6 = Calamus	28 = Rue
7 = Cassia	29 = Saffron
8 = Cedarwood	30 = Shittim or Acacia
9 = Cinnamon	31 = Spikenard
10 = Coriander	32 = Terebinth
11 = Cumin	33 = Wormwood
12 = Cypress	34 = Incense
13 = Dill	35 = Ointment
14 = Fir	36 = Odors
15 = Frankincense	37 = Perfume
16 = Galbanum	38 = Sweet Savors
17 = Henna or Camphire	39 = Spices
18 = Hyssop	40 = Embalming Oils
19 = Juniper	41 = Anointing Oil
20 = Mint or Peppermint	42 = Oils of Joy
21 = Mustard Seed	43 = Ess'l Oils by Context
22 = Myrrh	44 = Olive Oil

TABLE FIVE . . . Books that Mention Oils cont'd

Genesis   3, 12, 22, 32, 33, 38, 39, 40, 41, 44

Exodus   6, 7, 9, 10, 15, 16, 18, 22, 24, 30, 34, 35, 37, 38, 41, 44

Leviticus   8, 15, 18, 34, 36, 38, 41, 44

Numbers   1, 5, 8, 10, 15, 18, 34, 38, 41, 44

Deuteronomy 30, 34, 41, 44

Joshua   32

Judges   8, 32, 41

Ruth   41

I Samuel   34, 41

II Samuel   8, 14, 32, 41, 44

I Kings   8, 12, 14, 18, 19, 32, 39, 41, 43, 44

II Kings   8, 14, 35, 39, 41, 44

I Chronicles 8, 43, 15, 32, 34, 35, 39, 44

II Chronicles 8, 14, 34, 39, 41, 44

Ezra   8, 38, 44

Nehemiah   15, 23, 25, 44

Esther   22, 36

Job   8, 19, 35

Psalms   1, 4, 7, 8, 18, 19, 22, 34, 35, 41, 42

Proverbs   1, 9, 22, 33, 35, 37, 42, 43, 44

Ecclesiastes 35

Song Solomon 1, 6, 8, 9, 12, 14, 15, 17, 22, 27, 35, 37, 38, 39

Appendix B

Catalogue of Apocryphal Citations for Essential Oils & Aromatic Plants

The *Old Testament Apocrypha* (or *Deutero-canonical Books* of the *Bible*) consists of fifteen books or letters composed between 300 B.C. and 100 A.D. They fill the gap between the book of Malachi (the last book of the Protestant *Old Testament*) and the Gospels of the *New Testament*. They were considered as scriptures by the early Christians and were included in the Catholic *Vulgate* (or *Common Bible*) translated by St. Jerome into Latin and published around 390 A.D.

The Jews, however, while considering them as legitimate sources of history and spiritual wisdom, never elevated them to the same status as the *Old Testament*.

In 1534 A.D., when Martin Luther published his German translation, he lumped these books under the title of "Apocrypha" (meaning "hidden") and stated "These books are not held equal to the sacred scriptures and yet are useful and good for reading."

The Catholic Church reacted strongly. In 1546 A.D. at the Council of Trent they declared: "Whoever did not recognize as sacred and canonical all the books of the *Vulgate*, including the so called Apocryphal books, would be anathema." In other words, you would be declared a heretic and be subject to excommunication.

The committee of Anglican theologians, gathered by King James to create an English translation, disagreed with Martin Luther and included the *Apocrypha* as an official part of the original *King James Version* of 1611. However, the public was beginning to have doubts. By 1626 copies of the KJV began to circulate omitting the *Apocrypha.*

There was controversy among Protestants over these books for the next two hundred years. Finally, in 1827 the British and Foreign *Bible* Society (BFBS) and the American *Bible* Society (ABS) announced that they would "henceforth exclude, in their printed copies of the *English Bible,* the circulation of those books, or parts of books, which are usually termed Apocryphal."

The Authorized King James Version

Therefore, the *Revised Authorized King James Version* published in 1881, which is the version of the KJV accepted by most Protestant churches today, does not contain these books. Thus, few Christians, outside of Catholics, are familiar with them.

Despite their disputed history, they have always been accepted as valid representations of the history and life of the Jews in the centuries just before and after Jesus. Some of these books were familiar to Christ and his followers. They are also valid sources of information on the use of essential oils in that time between *Old Testament* and *New Testament.* Hence, we have chosen to include a catalogue of oil references in this book from the *Apocrypha.*

One book is particularly interesting, containing much wisdom that is well worth reading. It was written between 195 - 171 B.C. by Ben Sirach and is called the "Book of Sirach," but is also called "Ecclesiasticus."

Sirach 38:4 says, "The Lord created medicines from

the earth, and a sensible man will not despise them."
Of course, the medicines of the earth are plants, and
the most potently healing gifts of the plant kingdom
are their oils.

There is also a set of writings called the "*New
Testament Apocrypha*," but these books have yet to be
accepted by any church authority as being canonical.
Therefore, we did not include their consideration in
this book.

Our research has found 68 Apocryphal references
to essential oils and/or aromatic plants and 11
species, including three plant varieties not found in
the KJV *Bible*. This Appendix contains five tables as
follows:

TABLE ONE-B
Essential Oils and/or Aromatic Plants
of the Old Testament Apocrypha (11 species)

TABLE TWO-B
Specific Apocryphal References to Essential Oils
and/or Aromatic Plants (19 citations)

TABLE THREE-B
General Apocryphal References to Essential Oils
and/or Aromatic Plants (38 citations)

TABLE FOUR-B
Books of the Apocrypha that Mention Essential
Oils and/or Aromatic Plants (14 Books)

NOTE that no "indirect references" to oils were
found in the *Apocrypha* so there are only four tables
instead of the five as found in Appendix A.

The references to oils and plants in this Appendix are of are of two types as defined in Appendix A:

> (1) Specific References
> (2) General References

The format of Table One-B is the same as Table One-A and is defined in Appendix A.

Books of the Old Testament Apocrypha

The fifteen books of the Apocrypha are as follows:

I Esdras

II Esdras

Tobit

Judith

Additions to Esther

Wisdom of Solomon

Sirach (also called Ecclesiasticus)

Baruch

Letter of Jeremiah

Prayer of Azariah

Susanna

Bel and the Dragon

Prayer of Manasseh

I Maccabees

II Maccabees

TABLE ONE-B

Essential Oils and/or Aromatic Plants
of the Old Testament Apocrypha
(11 Species)
(See Table Four-B for the Scriptural Citations)

1. *CAMEL'S THORN 1x
(Balsamum)
Grk. aspalanthus, meaning "sweet scented shrub."
Alhagi maurorum (A.= sweet; m. = manna)

2. CASSIA 1x   (<u>cas</u> . si. a)
(Oriental Cinnamon)
Heb. qiddah, meaning "amber," or qetsioth, meaning
"bark like cinnamon" Grk. kasia = acacia
    Cinnamomum cassia (C.= like cinnamon; c.=
       Greek name for trees resembling acacias)

3. CEDARWOOD 4x   (<u>cee</u> . dar. wood)
(Juniper)
Heb. erez, meaning "hard wood" Gr. kedros, mean-
    ing "resinous tree"
Cedrus atlantica (C.= true cedar; a.= of the Atlas
    Mountains of Greece)

4. CYPRESS 2x   (<u>sy</u> . press)
(Gopherwood, Oil Tree)
Heb. tirzah. Grk. kyparissos
Cupressus sempervirens (C.= cypress tree;
    s.= everlasting or always green)

5. FRANKINCENSE 2x　　　　　(<u>frank</u> . in. cents)
(Incense, Olibanum)

Heb. lebonah. Grk. olibanos. Old Lat. olibanum. All
derived from the Arabic. al luban, meaning "milk."
In Late Latin, the language used in the Vulgate
or original Catholic Bible, it became francum incen-
sum, meaning literally, "real, pure, or true incense,"
which is where the King James Bible translators
got the English expression "Frankincense" we use
today.

Boswellia carteri (B.= after Scottish botanist Dr.
John Boswell; c.= after British surgeon and
herbologist Dr. H.J. Carter who first identified
the species and brought samples to England.

6. GALBANUM　1x　　　　　(<u>gal</u> . ba. num)
(Galban)

Heb. chelbanah or khelbnah, meaning "fatness"
Ferula Gummosa (F.= the giant fennel, a rod, or a
walking stick; g.= gummy resin)

7. MYRRH　1x　　　　　(murr)
(Balm, Balsam, Bdellium, Ladanum, Stacte)

Heb. mor. Grk. smurna, smurnizo, or muron. All of
which mean "bitter" in both languages

Commiphora myrrha (C.= gum bearing; m.= bitter)

8. ONYCHA　1x　　　　　(<u>on</u> . i. keh)
(Benzoin, Friar's Balm, Frankincense of Java)

Heb. shechelet, from an Arabic word referring to
the "husks of wheat or barley"

Styrax benzoin (S.= fragrant gum; b.= incense
of Java)

9. *ROSE BAY or OLEANDER 4x   (<u>o</u>. lee. an. der)
(Jericho Rose, Rose Laurel, Rose of the Brook)
Lat. orodandrum = rhododendren
Nerium oleander (N.= dark color; o. = corrupted
form of the Latin word for rhododendren, to which
oleander is not related at all)

10. TEREBINTH 1x   (<u>ter</u>. a. binth)
(Turpentine Tree, Palestinian Oak)
Heb. elah or allah
Pistacia terebinthus var. palestina (P.= pistachio
   tree; t.= turpentine tree; p.=from Palestine

11. *TRUE ROSE 1x
(Rose of the Mountains, True Rose, Bulgarian Rose)
Rosa damascena/phoenicia (R.= true rose; d. =
from Damascus; p.= from Phoenicia (Phoenicia
was called Tyre in the Bible)

* Those marked with an asterisk are species not found in
the Bible. There are only three: Camel's Thorn, Rose Bay
(Oleander), and True Rose. Camel's Thorn was a popular
plant that yielded a gum from which oils were extracted and
ointments made both for their medicinal properties and their
sweet scent. Camel's Thorn resin was sometimes
described by the Jews of that time as "white like manna."
See Chapter Eight entitled "Roses of the Scriptures."

TABLE TWO-B

Specific Apocryphal References to Essential Oils and/or Aromatic Plants
(There are 19 Citations in this Table)
(Also see Table One-B)

CAMEL'S THORN (Alhagi Maurorum)
Sirach 24:15

CASSIA (Cinnamomum Cassia)
Sirach 24:15

CEDARWOOD (Cedrus atlantica)
I Esdras 4:48; 5:55
Sirach 24:13; 50:10

CYPRESS (Cupressus sempervirens)
Sirach 24:13; 50:10

FRANKINCENSE (Boswellia Carteri)
Sirach 24:15; 39:14

GALBANUM (Ferula gummosa)
Sirach 24:15

MYRRH (Commiphora myrrha)
Sirach 24:15

ONYCHA (Styrax benzoin)
Sirach 24:15

ROSE BAY or OLEANDER (Nerium oleander)
Wisdom of Solomon 2:8
Sirach 24:14; 39:13; 50:8

TEREBINTH (Pistacia terebinthus)
Sirach 24:16

TRUE ROSE (Rose Damascena)
2 Esdras 2:19

NOTE: In Third Maccabees there are three mentions of Frankincense, three mentions of Myrrh, and one mention of True Rose, which would have been 7 more references to plants that yield essential oils. But Third Maccabees was written much later than the other books of the Apocrypha and is considered part of the Pseudepigrapha. It was never considered canonical by any church. So these were not tabulated here, although some authorities do include it with the Apocrypha.

TABLE THREE-B

General Apocryphal References
To Essential Oils and/or Aromatic Plants
(There are 38 references cited in this Table)

INCENSE 15x

Tobit 6:16, 8:2
Judith 9:1
Wisdom of Solomon 18:21
Sirach 45:16; 49:1; 50:9
Baruch 1:10
Letter of Jeremiah 6:43
Prayer of Azariah 15
I Maccabees 1:55; 4:49, 50
II Maccabees 2:5; 10:3

ODORS 7x

I Esdras 1:12
II Esdras 6:44
Tobit 8:3
Sirach 24:15; 35:6; 45:16; 50:15

FRAGRANCES 4x

2 Esdras 6:44
Sirach 24:15; 39:14a, 14b

PERFUME 4x

2 Esdras 2:12
Additions to Esther 14:2
Wisdom of Solomon 2:7
Sirach 49:1

SCENTED OIL 4x

I Esdras 6:30
Sirach 38:11; 45:15
Susanna 17

OINTMENT 3x

Judith 10:13; 16:8
Susanna 17

AROMA 1x

Sirach 12:15

TABLE FOUR–B

Books of the Apocrypha that Mention Essential Oils and/or Aromatic Plants

Only two Apocryphal books contain no reference to oils and/or aromatic plants: Prayer of Manasseh; Bel and the Dragon. That's 13 out of 15 or 87%. The following tabulation indicates what the books contain by use of the following key:

1 = Camel's Thorn
2 = Cassia
3 = Cedarwood
4 = Cypress
5 = Frankincense
6 = Galbanum
7 = Myrrh
8 = Onycha
9 = Jericho Rose (Oleander)

10 = Terebinth
11 = True Rose
12 = Incense
13 = Odors
14 = Fragrances
15 = Perfume
16 = Scented Oil
17 = Ointment
18 = Aroma

I Esdras	3, 13, 16
II Esdras	11, 13, 14, 15
Tobit	12, 13
Judith	12, 17
Additions to Esther	15
Wisdom of Solomon	9, 12, 15
Sirach	1, 2, 3, 4, 5, 6, 7, 8, 9, 10, 12, 13, 14, 15, 16, 18
Baruch	12
Letter of Jeremiah	12
Prayer Azariah	12
Susanna	16, 17
I Maccabees	12
II Maccabees	12

Appendix C
Oils of Biblical Times
Not Mentioned in the Bible

Essential oils were an important and daily part of the lives of those living in Biblical times, yet the *Bible* is incomplete and vague about their usage. Primarily, this is because it was not the intent of *Bible* writers to discuss oils but to present the word of God in the historical context of the Jews and early Christians. Hence, the majority of Biblical references to oils are related to worship (as in Exodus) and quasi-religious ceremonies, such as the anointing of kings (as found in Samuel, Kings, and Chronicles) or such as burial and embalming (as found in Genesis and the Gospels).

Nevertheless, we are fortunate to find as many mentions of essential oils and aromatic plants in the *Bible* as we do. The truth is that not only were the 33 species of aromatic plants and oils identifiable from the *Bible* in use by the peoples of that time, there were many more. Most of the oils and fragrances commonly used for medicines and fragrances for deodorants, perfumes, and incenses around the homes and businesses were omitted from the *Bible* because their mention would not contribute to making their theological point.

To find what other oils were in use during Biblical times, one has to rely on archeological records of the Babylonians, Sumerians, Phoenicians, Egyptians, Persians, Arabians, and other cultures that surrounded and occupied the Holy Land at those times. One also has to rely on Greek sources, such as those of the great physician, Hippocrates, 460–377 B.C., and Roman sources, such as those of Pliny the Elder (Caius Plinius Secundus), a Roman naturalist who wrote between 23–79 A.D. and Pliny the Younger (Caius Plinius Caecilius Secundus), a historian who wrote between 62–114 AD. A most important source is the more than two dozen volumes by the most important Jewish historian of his time, Josephus (Joseph Ben Matthias) who lived 37–100 A.D.

In some cases, plants, such as Myrtle, Cypress, Terebinth, Juniper, Pine and Fir are mentioned in the *Bible* but not the fact that oils were extracted and used from these plants. These outside sources are valuable in confirming that these plants of the *Bible* were also sources of essential oils used by the people of Biblical times by both Jews and Gentiles.

Research into such sources would be a project of many years and, perhaps, a book unto itself. Therefore, we did not consult any of these directly but relied on indirect sources that reviewed or mentioned these works. Several *Bible* and secular encyclopedias were valuable resources in this regard.

Two excellent books, with bibliographies containing many ancient references, are *The Art of Aromatherapy* by Robert Tisserand and *Frankincense and Myrrh* by Martin Watt and Wanda Sellar. Another source is the book, *375 Essential Oils and Hydrosols* by Jeanne Rose. An excellent scholarly source is the book, *Plants of the Bible*, by A.W. Anderson, who digresses into a number of plants not mentioned in the scriptures. All four of these works are listed in the Bibliography.

Where's the Lemon Oil?

As a last comment, you will notice that citrus fruits, citrus trees or their oils are nowhere mentioned in the *Bible* nor are they to be found in any of the writings or records of other Middle Eastern cultures of Biblical times.

That is because citrus is of Chinese origin and was not known in Europe and the Middle East until around the tenth century A.D. (Note that one of the scientific names for the orange is "Citrus sinensis," which means "fruit from China" or "fruit from the Orient.")

In modern aromatherapy, citrus oils play major roles in the healing of body, mind, and soul. but such medicines were unknown to the people of the *Bible.*

TABLE ONE-C

Essential Oils and Aromatic Plants Used in Biblical Times but <u>Not</u> Mentioned in the Bible
(31 Species)

NOTE: In giving a Genus and Species, sometimes several species or varieties could have been named for the same plant.

Angelica	Angelica archangelica
Basil	Ocimum basilicum
Bisabol	Commiphora erythraea
Black Pepper	Piper nigrum
Blue Tansy	Tanacetum annum
* Camel's Thorn	Alhagi mourorum
Cardamon	Elettaria cardamomum
Caraway	Carum carvi
Celery Seed	Apium graveolens
Citronella	Cymbopogen nardus
Clove	Syzygium aromatica
Costus	Saussurea lappa
Elemi	Canarium luzonicum
Fennel	Feoniculum vulgare
Galanga	Alpina officinarium
Ginger	Zingiber officinale
Jasmine	Jasminum officionale
Lily	Anemone coronaria
Lotus	Nymphaea lotus
Marjoram	Origanum majorana
Mum	Chrysanthemum aurum
* Oleander (Jericho Rose)	Nerium oleander
Opopanax	Opopanax chironium
Roman Chamomile	Chamaemelum nobile
* Rose (True Rose)	Rosa damascena/phoenicia
Rosemary	Rosmarinus officinalis
Rosewood	Aniba rosaedora
Sage	Salvia officinalis
Spruce	Picea mariana
Thyme	Thymus vulgaris
White (Sweet) Flag	Typha agustata

* Mentioned in the Old Testament Apocrypha

Kyphi
An Egyptian Blend of Biblical Times

Kyphi (or kuphi) was a blend of oils used by Egyptians for thousands of years from before the time of Joseph and the Israelite captivity through *New Testament* times. It was used in religious rituals, for emotional clearing and for other purposes unknown. Its exact formula was a closely guarded secret of the temple priests. However, several lists of ingredients have been published as being the oils of Kyphi. Martin Watt and Wanda Seller (see Bibliography) give a formula for the oils of Kyphi as follows:

> 6 parts Frankincense
> 4 parts Onycha
> 4 parts Myrrh
> 2 parts Juniper
> 1 part Galanga
> 1 part Cinnamon
> 1 part Cedarwood
> 4 drops Lotus
> 4 drops Honey with some Raisins

It is interesting to note that honey was an ingredient in the ointments and cosmetics of Hebrew women. Robert Tisserand gives a different list of principal oils for the Kyphi blend in his book as follows:

> Calamus
> Cassia
> Cinnamon
> Peppermint
> Citronella
> Pistacia (Terebinth)
> Juniper
> Acacia (Shittim)
> Henna (Camphire)
> Cypress
> Myrrh and Raisins

Appendix D
Olive and Other Fatty Oils Of the Biblical Times

This appendix provides the documentation for the chapter entitled "Olive Oil—The Other Healing Oil of the *Bible.*" The most common oil of the *Bible* is olive (Olea europea). The word, oil, is found in the *Bible* 191 times, and, in almost every instance, the reference is to olive oil or to essential oils containing olive as part of the blend.

While it is primarily a fatty oil used for food, cooking, and burning in lamps, the "first" or "beaten" olive oil (Exodus 27:20; Leviticus 24:2; Numbers 28:5) also naturally contains the essential oils of the olive fruit along with the fatty oil of the hard seed. You can read about that in more detail in the chapter named above. What we present here are the Biblical citations to olive as an oil, as a tree, as a wood, as a fuel, as a food, and in other contexts.

The only other fatty oil sources mentioned in the *Bible* are almond and flax (or linseed). We know that other vegetable oils were used, such as castor bean, walnut, sesame seed, and pistachio nut, but none of these are mentioned in the *Bible.* Their usage would have been minor compared to the consumption of olive, which played major roles in a variety of aspects of Hebrew and early Christian life.

Flax seed and walnut oils deserve a comment here, inasmuch as they, like olive, contain healing properties when consumed. Both of these oils have been shown to be particularly rich in omega-3 fatty acids. According to an article in *Natural Medicine Alert* (January 2001) the best form of omega 3 is alpha linolenic acid (ALA). Flax seed (linseed) oil is 53% ALA while walnut is 10% ALA. Both rank in the top ten oils for this factor.

It has been shown that a difficiency of essential fatty acids, particularly omega-3 and 6, may contribute to degenerative illnesses and symptoms such as diabetes, eczema, psoriasis, acne, learning/behavioral disorders, impaired cognitive development, impaired nerve function, cardiovascular disease, obesity, arthritis, depression, vision problems, cartilage destruction, and cancer.

Conversely, a diet rich in these oils can help reverse the conditions listed above or prevent them. A diet rich in omega-3 and 6, such as found in flax seed and walnut, has also been correlated with increased longevity.

It seems that the diet of Biblical peoples included some items that would be considered well chosen health foods today—foods that have now been scientifically proven to promote health.

Olive oil is special among all oils. Unlike any other fatty oil of Biblical times, olive was especially recognized by God for sacred applications. (Exodus 30:24) It was, thus, set apart from all others.

TABLE ONE-D

Catalogue of Scriptural References to Olive and Other Fatty Oils And/or their Sources
(3 Species)

ALMOND 4x (Amagdalus communis)

(Aaron's Rod, Wake Tree)

Genesis 43:11
Exodus 17:20
Numbers 17:8
Ecclesiastes 12:5

FLAX or LINSEED 3x (Lininum usitatissimum)

Exodus 9:31
Isaiah 42:3
Hosea 2:5

OLIVE OIL (identified as Olive) 7x (Olea europaea)

Exodus 27:20; 30:24
Leviticus 24:2
Deuteronomy 8:8; 28:40;
II Kings 18:32
Micah 6:15

MOUNT OF OLIVES 12x
(Site of Gethsemane and many Olive Groves)

Matthew 21:1; 24:3; 26:30
Mark 11:1; 13:3; 14:26
Luke 19:29, 37; 21:37; 22:39
John 8:1
Acts 1:12

OLIVE OIL (inferred as Olive) 147x (Olea europaea)

Genesis 28:18; 35:14

Exodus 25:6; 29:2, 40; 35:8, 14, 28; 39:37

Leviticus 2:1, 2, 4, 5, 6, 7, 10, 16; 5:11; 6:15, 21; 7:10, 12a, 12b; 8:2, 10, 12, 30; 9:4; 14:10, 12, 15, 16a, 16b, 17, 18, 21, 24, 26, 27, 28, 29; 21:10, 12; 23:13; 24:2

Numbers 4:9, 16; 5:15; 6:15a, 15b; 7:13, 19, 25, 31, 37, 43, 49, 55, 61, 67, 73, 79; 8:8; 11:8; 15:4, 6, 9; 18:12; 28:5, 9, 13, 20, 28; 29:3, 9, 14

Deuteronomy 8:8; 11:14; 12:17; 14:23; 18:4; 28:40, 51

II Samuel 14:2

I Kings 17:12, 14, 16

II Kings 4:2, 6, 7

I Chronicles 9:29; 12:40; 27:28

II Chronicles 2:10, 15; 11:11; 31:5; 32:28

Ezra 3:7; 6:9; 7:22

Nehemiah 5:11; 10:37. 39; 13:5, 12

Proverbs 21:17

Jeremiah 31:12; 40:10

Ezekiel 16:13, 18, 19; 23:41; 27:17; 45:14, 24, 25; 46:5, 7, 11, 14, 15

Hosea 2:5, 8, 22

Joel 1:10; 2:19, 24

Haggai 1:11; 2:12

Matthew 25:3, 4, 8

Luke 16:6

Revelation 18:13

GARDEN OF GETHSEMANE 2x

(Which was an Olive Garden and Vineyard. "Gethsemane" means "Oil-Wine Press")

Matthew 26:36

Mark 14:32

OLIVE TREES, WOOD, FRUIT, etc. 33x

Genesis 8:11
Exodus 23:11
Deuteronomy 6:11; 24:20; 28:40
Joshua 24:13
Judges 9:8, 9; 15:5
I Samuel 8:14
I Kings 6:23, 31, 32, 33
II Kings 5:26
I Chronicles 27:28
Nehemiah 5:11; 8:15; 9:25
Job 15:33
Psalm 52:8; 128:3
Jeremiah 11:16
Hosea 14:6
Amos 4:9
Micah 6:15
Habakkuk 3:17
Zechariah 4:3, 11, 12
Romans 11:17, 24
James 3:12
Revelation 11:4

OIL USED FOR FOOD 25x

Exodus 29:2, 23
Leviticus 2:5; 6:21 15a, 15b; 7:10, 12a, 12b; 8.8; 9:4;
        11:8; 23:13; 28:5
Numbers 6:15; 28:9, 12
Deuteronomy 12:17; 14:23
Ezra 3:7
Nehemiah 13:5
Proverbs 21:17
Ezekiel 16:13
Hosea 2:5
Haggai 2:12

OIL USED FOR LAMPS 9X
Exodus 25:6; 35:8, 14, 28; 39:37
Numbers 4:16
Matthew 25:3, 4; 25:6

BEATEN OR FIRST OLIVE OIL (VIRGIN) 3x
Exodus 27:20
Leviticus 24:2
Numbers 28:5

BIBLE **OILS OF UNKNOWN SPECIES OR TYPE 10x**
Deuteronomy 32:13; 33:24
Job 29:6
Psalms 55:21; 109:18; 141:5
Proverbs 5:3
Ezekiel 32:14
Micah 6:7
Revelation 6:6

THE PRIESTS' DUE
Oil As A Part of the Temple Offerings, etc.

The priests and their families were to be supported solely by the tithes and offerings to the temples they served. This included a portion of the sacrificial oils, grains, spices, and animals for meat. Only the best and finest were to be offered. Hence, only fragrant, flavorful "first," or "beaten," olive oil was acceptable, and not the "second" or "pressed" oil that was flavorless and had no aroma. There are several references to the priests' due in the Bible. Here are a few:

Leviticus 2:3, 10
Deuteronomy 14:27-29; 18:3-8
Numbers 7
Nehemiah 12:44-47

Appendix E
Seventh Heaven

This appendix provides background information for those doing the *Bible* Oils Program (Chapter Fourteen) who want to include the 7th Heaven Kit of oils in the presentation. You may photocopy the table of specific oils contained in the 7th Heaven Kit to hand out at your program if you wish. The text contained here as explanatory notes for the idea of "Seventh Heaven," is not intended as a handout to the public. You may verbally express whatever parts of the following discussion you deem appropriate to your audience at the time. For those in your audience interested in more information on this, suggest that they purchase this book.

What is Seventh Heaven?

Even without knowing where the idea came from, we all know that "being in Seventh Heaven" is a state of supreme happiness, joy, bliss, ecstasy, or satisfaction. That much everyone knows. But where did this expression come from and does it have a basis in scripture?

The concept of "Seventh Heaven" originates from the secret teachings of the Jews that were intended to be passed on by word of mouth only. The concept was not supposed to appear in print. Originally, such knowledge was only to be shared with those deemed spiritually ready to receive it. However, references to it can be found in the Talmud (which was originally verbal) as well as in the *Pseudepigrapha*—a collection of Jewish and early Christian writings from 100 B.C. to 600 A.D. ("Pseudepigrapha" means "false writings." This is because all of the names of the given authors are known to be false and not the true writers.)

Seven levels of heaven (or degrees of awareness of God) was also an esoteric teaching of the Essenes, a colony of Jewish mystics who lived near the Dead Sea from approximately 100 B.C. to 100 A.D. Many Biblical scholars believe that Jesus may have studied and lived with the Essenes. Their teachings, as found in the Dead Sea Scrolls, are very similar to many of his own expressed during his brief three-year ministry.

The concept of Seventh Heaven was this: In order to reach God, one ascends through seven "levels" or "rings" of consciousness (or spiritual awareness) with the top, or seventh level, being total awareness of or complete communion with God, himself.

Jesus and Seventh Heaven

Jesus was, no doubt, aware of the these teachings as were his disciples, since most Jews had at least heard of the idea by *New Testament* times. For some reason, however, they were never included in the Gospels. Because they were supposed to be "secret" and not made available to the public in general, perhaps the Gospel writers didn't mention the idea out of respect for the notion that they were to be shared only with select persons of sufficient spiritual development to understand and make use of the concept.

The only place the concept appears explicitly in the *Old Testament* and *New Testament* is in II Corinthians where St. Paul comments:

> "I knew a man in Christ . . . caught up to the Third Heaven . . . How he was caught up into paradise and heard unspeakable things." (II Corinthians 12:2, 4)

Paul, of course, being a well-educated Jewish insider, would have been well aware of the confidentiality of such teachings and did not explain nor elaborate on the idea in his letter. He was apparently writing to people who would have known about the idea of seven levels of heaven already, and if they didn't, then it was not for him to explain or expound on the concept in a public letter. His reference to "unspeakable things" is probably a reference to the esoteric, secret, or mystical nature of such experiences, which were to be shared with only a select few.

Another place in the *Bible* that may be referring to "seventh heaven," or the concept of "seven levels of spiritual awareness," is described symbolically in Revelation.

"And being turned I saw seven candlesticks, and in the midst of the seven candlesticks one like unto the Son of Man. . . And he had in his right hand seven stars . . . And he laid his right hand upon me, saying unto me, Fear not: I am the first and the last: I am he that liveth, and was dead; and, behold, I am alive for evermore Amen; and have the keys of hell and of death. Write the things which thou hast seen, and the things which are, and the things which shall be hereafter; The mystery of the seven stars which thou sawest in my right hand, and the seven golden candlesticks. The seven stars are the angels of the seven churches: and the seven candlesticks which thou sawest are the seven churches." (Revelation 1:12-13, 17-20)

Revelation continues with more references to seven stars (2:1; 3:1), seven candlesticks (2:1), seven spirits of God (3:1; 4:5; 5:6), seven lamps (4:5) , seven eyes (5:6), seven angels (8:2, 6), seven trumpets (8:2, 6), seven thunders (10:3, 4), and seven seals (5:1, 5). Some scholars have interpreted these metaphors as representations of the "seventh heaven" concept of levels of ascension to God.

John, the author of Revelation, was almost certainly familiar with the esoteric concept of "seventh heaven." John was clearly in communion with God at the highest levels. If there were actually seven heavens, he would certainly have experienced them all and would have realized their existence first hand.

In Revelation 1:19 we see that John writes his observations of the seven stars, seven seals, etc. at the request of Christ himself. Apparently, with the publishing of the Book of Revelation around 100 A.D., the teachings were no longer to be kept in such secret. However, even with John's writings made public, the symbolic language he used still shrouds the teachings in secrecy and mysticism to be understood only by a few with the spiritual insight to interpret his words.

There is more to the concept of "seventh heaven" than the mere intellectual idea of it. That much you have been given here in this Appendix. The full teaching, which was the real secret, included detailed instructions on how to actually reach and experience each of the seven levels, what to expect at each step of the way, what obstacles or difficulties may appear, and how to deal with them such that your journey to God might be successful.

Secret Teachings of Jesus

Jesus spent a great deal of time in private instruction with his twelve. They were all individually selected, spiritually advanced disciples. Jesus taught them things that were never made public in any of their writings. (John 21:25) Esoteric or "hidden" teachings were actually a regular part of Jesus' manner of speech which was often disguised in parables, symbols, and metaphors.

When he spoke publicly, his messages were never expected nor intended to be understood by everyone. He spoke in parables so that those who were not ready to accept the truth, and unable to benefit from it, would not grasp it. Christ's phrase, "He that hath ears to hear, let him hear," is found seven times in the Gospels. The same thought is expressed eight times in Revelation (2:7, 11, 17, 29; 3:6, 13, 22; 13:9).

Did Jesus teach the idea of passing through seven levels to reach God? We don't know if he did or not. "Seventh Heaven," as a concept, was known and understood by many people of Christ's day. That much we do know. The purpose of this Appendix is merely to explain where the expression originated. So now you know.

Pages You May Photocopy for Your Program

• Appendix F, (pp. 280-299) contains pages you may photocopy as handouts on oils of ancient scripture for your audience when you do a *Bible* Oils Program. They are not to be sold or distributed outside of programs that you personally do.

• If you include the Seventh Heaven Kit of Essential Oils in your *Bible* Oils Program, (See Chapter 14) you may want to give your participants a handout for seventh heaven, too. (pp. 277-279)

• Permission is hereby granted for you to photocopy pages 276-299 of this book for free handouts at a *Bible* Oils Program. The notices at the bottoms of all of these pages are to remain as a legible part of the duplicates you distribute at your programs.

• You do not have permission to photocopy the foregoing discussion in this Appendix, or any other portion of this book than the pages specified in this notice, but you may verbally share any and all of the information contained in this book with whomever you choose.

• You have permission to cover this notice when you make duplicates for your programs and place here, instead, appropriate information about yourself and/or your group. This would include names, addresses, phone numbers, and any other information you would like for your participants to have after attending your *Bible* Oils Program.

THE 7th HEAVEN KIT
of Essential Oils

The phrase, "Seventh Heaven," is a spiritual concept held by Jews in Christ's time. Discussions of the idea can be found in the *Talmud*, the *Pseudepigrapha*, and the *Dead Sea Scrolls*. It concerns levels of spiritual achievement—Seventh being the highest state of divine communion. The *Bible* (via St. Paul) alludes to the idea as follows: "I knew a man in Christ . . caught up to the Third Heaven . . . How he was caught up into paradise and heard unspeakable things." II Corinthians 12:2, 4.

In the table below, oils denoted by asterisks (*) are mentioned in the *Bible*. Those denoted by (†) were oils used in Biblical times, but not mentioned in the *Bible*. Information on the contents and benefits of the seven blends listed here is adapted from the *Essential Oils Desk Reference* (EODR).

The Seven Oils of 7th Heaven

1. DREAM CATCHER™
Contents: *Sandalwood, †Blue Tansy, *Juniper, Bergamot, †Black Pepper
Benefits: May help open the mind and enhance dreams and visualization, promoting a greater potential for realizing your dreams and staying on your path. Also protects from negative dreams that might cloud your vision.

2. GATHERING™
Contents: *Galbanum, *Frankincense, *Sandalwood, †Rose, Lavender, *Cinnamon, †Spruce, Ylang Ylang, Geranium.
Benefits: May help overcome the bombardments of chaotic energy that alters our focus and takes us off our path toward higher achievements. May help bring people together on a physical, emotional, and spiritual level for greater focus and clarity. It may also help one stay focused, grounded, and clear in gathering one's potential for self-improvement.

Available from: Care Publications, RR 4, Box 646, Marble Hill, MO 63764
(573) 238-4846 • <care@clas.net> • Price: $19.95 + 6 s&h

3. AWAKEN™

<u>Contents:</u>This oil is a blend of blends as follows: JOY™, FORGIVENESS™, PRESENT TIME™, DREAM CATCHER™ and HARMONY™ which combined contain the following single oils: †Angelica, Bergamot, †Blue Tansy, *Frankincense, Geranium, Helichrysum, *Hyssop, †Jasmine, *Juniper, Lavender, Lemon, Mandarin, Melissa, Neroli, Orange, Palmarosa, †Roman Chamomile, †Rose, †Rosewood, *Sandalwood, †Spruce, and Ylang Ylang.

<u>Benefits</u>: Not intended to awaken us as in being tired or sleepy, but to awaken our spiritual awareness and consciousness of our true inner selves. Helps to bring one to an inner knowing in order to make changes and desirable transitions assisting to reach one's highest potential.

4. HUMILITY™

<u>Contents</u>: Frankincense, Rose, Rosewood, Ylang Ylang, Geranium, Melissa, Spikenard, Myrrh, Neroli, †Sesame Seed

<u>Benefits</u>: Having humility and forgiveness helps us to heal ourselves as well as our earth. (II Chronicles 7:14) Humility is necessary in obtaining forgiveness and is the only way to build a closer relationship with God. Through the frequency and fragrance of this blend, you may find that special place where your own healing may begin.

5. INSPIRATION™

<u>Contents</u>: *Frankincense, *Cedarwood, †Spruce, †Rosewood, *Sandalwood, *Myrtle, Mugwort

<u>Benefits</u>: May bring us closer to our spiritual connections. While composed almost entirely of Biblical oils, cedarwood and spruce were also used by Native Americans to increase spirituality, enhancing prayer and inner awareness. It is supportive of healthy bladder and kidney function.

---

6. SACRED MOUNTAIN™

<u>Contents</u>: †Spruce, *Fir, *Cedarwood, Ylang Ylang

<u>Benefits</u>: When we go into the mountains, our bodies feel recharged, our breath refreshed, and our minds calmed from the fragrance of shrubs and forest. Extracted from conifer trees, this blend represents the sacred feeling of the mountains. It stimulates feelings of protection, strength, grounding, empowerment, and security. It is supportive of the respiratory system.

7. WHITE ANGELICA™

<u>Contents</u>: Ylang Ylang, †Rose, Melissa, *Sandalwood, Geranium, †Spruce, *Myrrh, *Hyssop, Bergamot, †Rosewood, *Almond.

<u>Benefits</u>: Some of these oils were used in ancient times to increase intensity and size of the torus or aura (electric field) around the body. Its frequency neutralizes negative energy. It is calming, soothing, strengthening, and protective. It brings a feeling of security and a sense of spiritual wholeness. This oil is often used when doing emotional releases with people or when in any environment where negativity of any kind may be encountered, including the presence of demonic possessions.

Sesquiterpenes are common essential oil constituents that carry oxygen to the brain. The four oils of the world containing the highest percents of sesquiterpenes are as follows: Cedarwood 98%, Vetiver 97%, Spikenard 93%, and Sandalwood 90%. Cedarwood, Spikenard, and Sandalwood are Biblical oils, all of which are contained in the 7th Heaven collection of oils given above.

Available from: Care Publications, RR 4, Box 646, Marble Hill, MO 63764
(573) 238-4846 • <care@clas.net> • Price: $19.95 + 6 s&h

Appendix F
Principal Oils
of Ancient Scripture

In **Proverbs 21:20** we read: "There is treasure to be desired and oil in the dwelling of the wise." Question: Why would the possession of oil in one's house be a sign of wisdom? At least 33 different essential oils or aromatic oil-producing plants are mentioned in the *Bible* (12 of them are discussed in this Appendix plus cinnamon and calamus.)

The word "oil" is mentioned 191 times in the *Bible*. While "olive oil" is specifically mentioned only 7 times there are 147 instances where it can be inferred. (See Appendix D.) Olive oil was not only a food, but was burned in lamps for light and used as a base for blending other oils for religious or medicinal purposes.

"Incense" is mentioned 68 times in the *Bible*. In 54 of these the oils of frankincense, myrrh, galbanum, and onycha are indicated. In other instances, the Hebrew word translated into English as "incense" was "lebonah," which is actually frankincense. In only eight of the instances where incense is mentioned are the oils in the formula not identifiable.

In **Psalm 45:7-8, Proverbs 27:9, Isaiah 61:3** and **Hebrews 1:9** we read of "The Oil of Joy" or "Gladness" and how oils "rejoice the heart." Essential oils are also referred to in the *Bible* as "fragrances," "odors," "ointments," "aromas," "perfumes" or "sweet savors."

There are over 600 references to essential oils and/or the aromatic plants from which they were extracted in the *Bible*. (See Appendix C for a complete list.)

The fourteen principal oils of the *Bible* are listed below in order of the most frequently mentioned (Myrrh 156x) to the least mentioned (Rose of Sharon 3x).

FOURTEEN PRINCIPAL OILS OF THE BIBLE

1. MYRRH
Mentioned 18x directly + 138x indirectly = 156x
Chemistry: Sesquiterpenes-62%

2. FRANKINCENSE
Mentioned 22x directly + 59x indirectly = 81x
Chemistry: Monoterpenes-42%, Sesquiterpenes-8%

3. CEDARWOOD
Mentioned 5x directly + 65x as trees/wood = 70x
Chemistry: Sesquiterpenes-98%

4. CINNAMON
Mentioned 4x directly + 65x indirectly = 69x
Chemistry: Aldehydes, Phenylpropanoids

5. CASSIA
Mentioned 3x directly + 65x indirectly = 68x
Chemistry: Aldehydes, Esters, Phenylpropanoids

6. CALAMUS
Mentioned 3x directly + 65x indirectly = 68x
Chemistry: Phenylpropanoids

Available from: Care Publications, RR 4, Box 646, Marble Hill, MO 63764
(573) 238-4846 • <care@clas.net> • Price: $19.95 + 6 s&h

7. GALBANUM
Mentioned 1x directly + 54x indirectly = 55x
Chemistry: Monoterpenes-70%, Sesquiterpenes-15%

8. ONYCHA (FRIAR'S BALM/BENZOIN)
Mentioned 1x directly = 54x indirectly = 55x
Chemistry: Phenylpropanoids, Aldehydes

9. SPIKENARD (NARD)
Mentioned 7x directly + 10x indirectly = 17x
Chemistry: Sesquiterpenes-93%

10. HYSSOP
Mentioned 12x directly = 12x
Chemistry: Phenolic ketones 50%, Monoterpenes-30%, Sesquiterpenes 5-10%

11. SANDALWOOD (ALOES)
Mentioned 5x directly = 5x
Chemistry: Sesquiterpenes-90%

12. MYRTLE
Mentioned 6x directly = 6x
Chemistry: Monoterpenes-25%, Sesquiterpenes-9%

13. CYPRESS
Mentioned 1x directly + 4x indirectly = 5x
Chemistry: Monoterpenes-28%, Sesquiterpenes-25%

14. ROSE OF SHARON (CISTUS/ROCK ROSE)
Mentioned 1x directly + 2x indirectly = 3x
Chemistry: Monoterpenes-54%

UNIQUE CHEMISTRY OF BIBLICAL OILS:

Biblical oils contain three main classes of compounds: Sesquiterpenes, Monoterpenes and Phenylpropanoids. There are more than 10,000 varieties of sesquiterpenes, more than 2,000 varieties of monoterpenes, and hundreds of phenylpropanoids. Phenylpropanoids are antiseptic and cleanse receptor sites. Sesquiterpenes are oxygenating, mood elevating, and deprogram miswritten codes in the DNA. Monoterpenes are hostile to microbes and reprogram cells with correct information.

Sesquiterpenes are in: Cedarwood 98%, Spikenard 93%, Sandalwood 90%, Myrrh 62%, Galbanum 30%, Cypress 25%, Hyssop 20%, Myrtle 9%, Frankincense 8%. As for Monoterpenes, the main one is alpha Pinene found in: Rose of Sharon 50%, Galbanum 45%, Frankincense 40%, Cypress 28%, Myrtle 25%, Spikenard 2%. While sesquiterpenes and alpha pinene are spiritually elevating their oxygenating capabiities create an environment that makes it difficult for cancer cells to survive. They are also strong supporters of the immune system and boost the body's natural defenses.

Phenylpropanoids are found in: Calamus, Cinnamon, Galbanum, Onycha, and Spikenard. Phenols cleanse cellular receptor sites and promote hormonal balance and healthy bodily function. Modern research has found Cinnamon to be as effective against certain bacteria as Penicillin and Ampicillin. (2nd ed. EODR, p. 411) The Monoterpene, Camphene, found in Galbanum and Rose of Sharon, is virucidal, can cleanse the circulatory system, and also cleanses receptor sites. Thus, the Oils of the *Bible* serve us on all levels: Spiritual, Emotional, Mental, and Physical.

Available from: Care Publications, RR 4, Box 646, Marble Hill, MO 63764
(573) 238-4846 • <care@clas.net> • Price: $19.95 + 6 s&h

(Read **Exodus 30:22-31**)

TWO BLENDS OF BIBLICAL OILS

EXODUS II™ (Oil Blend)

Ingredients listed in order of the relative amounts contained in the blend (See 2nd edition of EODR pp. 96-97.)

1. Cassia   (*Cinnamomum cassia*)   Exodus 30:24
2. Hyssop   (*Hyssopus officinalis*)   Exodus 12:22
3. Frankincense (*Boswellia carteri*)   Exodus 30:34
4. Spikenard   (*Nardostachys jatamansi*) Song 1:12
5. Galbanum   (*Ferula gumosa*)   Exodus 30:34
6. Myrrh   (*Comiphora myrrha*)   Exodus 30:23
7. Cinnamon   (*Cinnamomum verum*)   Exodus 30:23
8. Calamus*   (*Acorus calamus*)*   Exodus 30:23
     Carrier Oil: Olive

 * Calamus is not available alone, only in this blend. The effective action of this oil blend against a variety of microbes is similar to that of another oil blend called Thieves™, which also contains cinnamon oil.

3 WISE MEN™ (Oil Blend)

Ingredients listed in order of the relative amounts contained in the blend (See 2nd edition EODR p. 124.)

1. Sandalwood   (*Santalum album*)   John 19:39
2. Juniper   (*Juniperus osteosperma*)   Job 30:4
3. Frankincense (*Boswellia carteri*)   Matthew 2:11
4. Myrrh   (*Comiphora myrrha*)   Mark 15:23
5. Spruce*   (*Picea mariana*)   *Not in *Bible*
     Carrier Oil: Almond

 * Spruce is not mentioned in the *Bible*, but was used during Biblical times. Spruce, Frankincense, and the other oils of a blend called Valor™, were used by Roman soldiers as emotional support to boost their courage before battle.

SELECTED OILS OF ANCIENT SCRIPTURE

1. ALOES/SANDALWOOD
Santalum album   **Family: Sandalaceae**

• Scriptures: Numbers 24:6; Psalms 45:8

Proverbs 7:17; Song of Solomon 4:14;

John 19:39

• Source: Wood of the tree

• Chemistry: Sesquiterpenes 90%: Sesquiterpene alcohols: Santalols; Sesquiterpene aldehydes; Carbonic Acid

• Ancient Uses: Assistance in Meditation; Aphrodisiac; Embalming

• Modern Uses: Sandalwood contains the fourth highest concentration of sesquiterpenes of all the oils-(90%). Sesquiterpenes deprogram misinformation and carry oxygen at a cellular level. Used for skin care, enhances deep sleep (stimulating release of melatonin); supportive of female reproductive and endocrine systems; has been applied for urinary tract infections.

• Applications: Diffuse, apply topically, ingest orally, burn in incense.

• Aloes/Sandalwood oil is found In:

7th Heaven Kit (Dream Catcher™, Gathering™, Inspiration™, White Angelica™, Awaken™) Harmony™, 3 Wise Men™

Available from: Care Publications, RR 4, Box 646, Marble Hill, MO 63764
(573) 238-4846 • <care@clas.net> • Price: $19.95 + 6 s&h

2. CASSIA
Cinnamomum cassia
Family: Lauraceae (laurel)

• Scriptures: Exodus 30:24; Psalms 45:8
Ezekiel 27:19

• Source: Bark of the tree

• Chemistry: Phenylpropanoids, Cinnamaldehyde, Benzaldehyde, Cinamyl Acetate,
Cinnamic Alcohol

• Ancient Uses: Ingredient in Moses' Holy
Anointing Oil.

• Modern Uses: Immune system builder and
supportive of the body's natural defenses.
Applications: Diffuse, topically, orally, incense

• Cassia oil is also found in Exodus II™

CINNAMON
Cinnamomum verum
Family: Lauraceae (laurel)

• Scriptures: Exodus 30:23   Proverbs 7:17
Song of Solomon 4:14; Revelation 18:13

• Source: Bark of the tree

• Chemistry: Cinnamaldehyde; Hydroxy-
cinnamaldehyde; Esters; Phenols:
Phenylpropanoids, Coumarins

• Ancient Uses: Holy Anointing Oils. Perfume.

• Modern Uses: Coumarins are antibacterial and antiviral phenols. Combined with the aldehydes, cinnamon is one of the most powerful antibacterial oils of all (tested against antibiotics). Has been applied to Tropical diseases and typhoid; can be sexually stimulating (aldehydes do that). Coumarins and Phenols cleanse receptor sites.

• Applications:Diffuse in blends (Thieves), topically, orally, incense

• Cinnamon bark oil is found in:
7th Heaven Kit (Gathering™)   Exodus II™
Abundance™, Christmas Spirit™, Thieves™

CALAMUS
Acorus calamus   **Family: Araceae (flag)**

• Scriptures: Exodus 30:23, Song Solomon 4:13-14, Ezekiel 27:19

• Source: Stems and leaves

• Chemistry: Phenylpropanoids

• Ancient Uses: Holy anointing oil, perfumes, incense. An aromatic stimulant and tonic for digestive system.

• Modern Uses: Relaxing to muscles, soothes inflammation, supportive of respiratory system, helps clear kidney congestion after intoxication.

• Applications: Topically over abdomen, orally, incense.

Calamus cont'd on next page . . .

Available from: Care Publications, RR 4, Box 646, Marble Hill, MO 63764
(573) 238-4846 • <care@clas.net> • Price: $19.95 + 6 s&h

Calamus cont'd

• Calamus oil is found in:
Exodus II™ (Calamus not available as a single oil. Only available in Exodus II)

3. CEDARWOOD
Cedrus atlantica   **Family: Pinaceae**

• Scriptures: Leviticus 14:4, 6, 49, 51, 52
Numbers 19:6

• Source: From bark of trees

• Chemistry: Sesquiterpenes 98% (the highest of any oil) Sesquiterpene alcohols; Sesquiterpene ketones; Other Sesquiterpenes

• Ancient Uses: Cleansing of lepers, ritual cleansing after touching a dead body or anything else considered "unclean," ritual cleansing from evil spirits, cosmetics, embalming, skin problems, various medicines, calming effects. This may be the first and most ancient of the distilled oils inasmuch as Chinese, Sumerians and Egyptians were using Oil of Cedarwood for embalming, disinfecting, hygienic, and other purposes more than 5,000 years ago. Mentioned on a Babylonian tablet dated 1800 B.C.

• Modern Uses: Insect repellent, hair loss, tuberculosis, bronchitis, gonorrhea, skin disorders (acne, psoriasis). Cedarwood is highest known oil in sesquiterpenes (98%) which can deprogram misinformation and bring oxygen to cellular levels. Enhances deep sleep (melatonin stimulant), emotional releases, promotes mental clarity.

• Applications: Diffuse, topically, orally, incense.

• Cedarwood oil is also found in:
7th Heaven Kit (Inspiration™, Sacred
Mountain™) and Brain Power™

FOR BIBLE OILS PROGRAM
TAKE A 15 MINUTE BREAK AT THIS POINT

4. CYPRESS
Cupressus sempervirens
Family: Cupressaceae

• Scriptures: Genesis 6:14; Isaiah 44:14; 44:14;
I Kings 9:11; Song of Solomon 1:17

• Source: From branches

• Chemistry: Monoterpenes: alpha Pinene;
Sesquiterpenes: Sesquiterpene alcohols;
Diterpene alcohols

• Ancient Uses: Arthritis, laryngitis, reducing
scar tissue, cramps. Cypress oil is mentioned in
a Babylonian tablet dating 1800 B.C.

• Modern Uses: Supportive of the cardiovascular
system (increases circulation, strengthens blood
capillaries, controls hemorrhages and nose
bleeds, relieves acute chest discomfort), emotionally beneficial: eases feeling of loss, promotes
feelings of security and grounding; supportive of
women during menstruation and menopause.
Monoterpenes reprogram cellular memory with
correct information thus promoting permanent
healings at a cellular level. Cypress also pro-

Cypress cont'd

motes production of leucocytes (white blood cells) which boosts the body's natural defenses.

• Applications: Massage along spine, on arm pits, on feet, heart and chest.

• Cypress oil is found in:
Aroma Seiz™ (for muscle cramps), Aroma Life™ (for chest pains), R.C.™ (respiratory congestion)

5. GALBANUM
Ferula gummosa   **Family: Apiaceae (parsley)**

• Scriptures: **Exodus 30:34-36**

• Source: Resins in stems and branches

• Chemistry: Monoterpenes: alpha Pinene, camphene, limonene, myrcene, carvone;
Sesquiterpene alcohols; Esters, Coumarins

• Ancient Uses: Holy anointing oils, various medicines, perfume, spiritually uplifting yet grounding, pain relief, spasms and cramps, diuretic.

• Modern Uses: Abscesses, acne, asthma, chronic coughs, cramps, indigestion, muscular aches and pains, scar tissue, wrinkles, wounds, emotionally balancing. Monoterpenes reprogram cellular memory thus promoting permanent healing. Coumarins are antiseptic phenols with an earthy smell like freshly mown hay or grass.

• Application: Topically, orally

• Galbanum oil is found in:
7th Heaven Kit (Gathering™) and Exodus II™

6. FRANKINCENSE
Boswellia carteri   **Family: Burseraceae**

• Scriptures: Exodus 30:34; Leviticus 2:1, 1, 15, 16; 5:11; 6:15; 24:7: **Numbers** 5:15; **16:46-50** (Aaron stops a plague); I Chron 9:29 Nehemiah 13:5, 9; Song of Solomon 3:6; 4:6, 14 **Isaiah 59:20; 60:3, 6** (These verses from Isaiah prophesy the gifts of the wise men) Isaiah 66:3; Jeremiah 6:20; 17:26; 41:5 (NOTE: these six references from Isaiah and Jeremiah, are translated as "incense" in the KJV. However, the Hebrew in all cases is "lebonah" which is frankincense. **Matthew 2:11** (Three wise men's visit) Revelations 18:13

• Source: Oleo-gum-resin from the trunks and limbs of the tree. Note that Myrrh is also a gum resin from a desert tree of the same family— Burseraceae—as was the Balm of Gilead.

• Chemistry: Monoterpenes: alpha Pinene, Limonene, Sesquiterpenes 8%; Terpene alcohols: Borneol

• Ancient Uses: Holy Anointing Oil, a cure-all, used to enhance meditation and elevate spiritual consciousness, thought to assist one in the transition of death, used for embalming, and perfume. Frankincense was used to anoint the newborn sons of kings and priests, which may have been why it was brought to the baby Jesus. Frankincense is mostly monoterpenes which, as an anointing oil, embraces God's image in us (Genesis 1:26). (See Chapter 2, pp. 27-31)

Available from: Care Publications, RR 4, Box 646, Marble Hill, MO 63764
(573) 238-4846 • <care@clas.net> • Price: $19.95 + 6 s&h

Frankincense cont'd

• Modern Uses: Monoterpenes reprogram cellular memory thus promoting permanent healing; helps maintain normal cellular regeneration; cancer, depression, allergies, headaches, bronchitis, herpes, tonsillitis, typhoid, warts, brain damage, massive head injuries, stimulates body's production of white corpuscles (immune builder), expectorant. Used in commercial fragrances: Old Spice™ (Shulton), Cinnabar™ and Youth Dew™ (Estee Lauder).

• Application: Diffuse, topically, orally, incense.

• Frankincense oil is found in:
7th Heaven Kit (Gathering™, Humility™, Inspiration™, Awaken™ (Forgiveness™, Harmony™)), Exodus II™, 3 Wise Men™, Abundance™, Acceptance™, Brain Power™, Trauma Life™, Valor™

7. **HYSSOP**
Hyssopus officinalis
Family: Lamiaceae (mint)

• Scriptures: **Exodus 12:22**   Leviticus 14:4, 6, 49, 51, 52; Numbers 19:6, 18; I Kings 4:33; **Psalms 51:7; John 19:29** ; Hebrews 9:19

• Source: Stems and Leaves

• Chemistry: Phenolic ketones 50%; Monoterpenes 20-30%; Sesquiterpenes 5-10%; Phenylpropanoids, Ethers 1-3%

• Ancient Uses: Spiritually cleansing, help for focusing mind in meditation, purification from sin, addictions and destructive habits; various medicines, respiratory relief, decongestant, expectorant. repeller of evil spirits (During the Passover, the Israelites struck the posts and lintels of their doorways with an branch of hyssop releasing its aromatic oils, along with the lamb's blood, as protection from the death angel.) During his last moments on the cross, Jesus was offered a sponge with sour wine extended with a fragrant branch of hyssop. Why hyssop? Crucifixion is death by slow suffocation as one's lungs gradually fill up with fluid. Breathing the scent of hyssop may have been offered by ladies of mercy to those dying by crucifixion to help ease their congestion and provide some relief both physically and emotionally.

• Modern Uses: Monoterpenes reprogram miswritten information in the DNA and thus promote permanent healing at a cellular level. Hyssop has been used to relieve anxiety, arthritis, asthma, respiratory infections, parasites, sore throats, cuts and wounds. Metabolizes fat, increases perspiration, detoxifying, and emotionally balancing. Lamiaceae is the same family of plants as many of the Raindrop Oils: Basil, Marjoram, Oregano, Thyme, and Peppermint.

• Applications: Diffuse, topically, orally

• Hyssop oil is found in:
7th Heaven Kit (White Angelica™, Awaken™)
Harmony™, Exodus II™, Relieve It™,
Immupower™

---

8. MYRRH
Commiphora myrrha   **Family: Burceraceae**

• Scriptures: Genesis 37:25; 43:11; Exodus 30:23; **Esther 2:12;** Psalms 45:8; Proverbs 7:17 (Also in Exodus 30:34 as "Stacte"); Song Solomon 1:13; 3:6; 4:6, 14; 5:1, 5, 13; Matthew 2:11; 26:7, 9, 12; Mark 14:3, 4; **Mark 15:23**; Luke 7:37, 38, 46; 23:56; John 11:2; 12:3, 5; 19:39

• Source: Oleo-gum-resin from the trunks and limbs of the tree. Note that Frankincense is also a gum resin from a desert tree of the same family—Burseraceae—as was the Balm of Gilead.

• Chemistry: Sesquiterpenes 62%: Sesqui-terpene furonics; Sesquiterpene Ketones; Hydrocarbons; Aldehydes.

• Ancient Uses: Pregnant mothers anointed them-selves for protection against infectious diseases and to elevate feelings of well-being. They also believed it would protect their unborn children from generational curses. (Exodus 20:5, 34:7; Numbers 14:18; Deuteronomy 5:9) Diffused and inhaled during labor to reduce anxiety and facili-tate calmness and massaged on perineum to facili-tate stretching. Used after childbirth to prevent or remove abdominal stretch marks. Customarily used on umbilical cords of newborn to protect navel from infection, which symbolically is meant to cut off generational curses inherited from ances-tors. It may have been for all of these uses that Myrrh was brought to Mary and baby Jesus.

Also used in ancient times for skin conditions, oral hygiene, embalming, and as an insect repellent. Egyptians carried cones of fat on their heads containing Myrrh that would melt in the desert heat and keep their bodies bathed in Myrrh and other oils.

Myrrh has always been a popular fixing oil, from ancient times to the present, to prolong the life of the fragrances in other oils. Hence, it was blended with so many perfumes and ointments in Biblical times that in the Gospels the Greek word for myrrh, "muron," was sometimes translated as "ointment" without revealing that its content included myrrh. (See Chapter Ten.)

• Modern Uses: Antiseptic, balancing to thyroid and endocrine system, supports immune system. Bronchitis, diarrhea, thrush in babies, vaginal thrush, athletes foot, ring worm, viral hepatitis, chapped skin, wrinkles. Emotionally releasing. Sesquiterpenes deprogram miswritten information on the DNA at a cellular level, thus promoting permanent healings. As in ancient times, myrrh is still used as a fixative to extend the fragrances of other scents.

It is used in many perfumes such as Alliage™ (Estee Lauder), Matchbelli™ (Matchbelli) and LeSport™ (St. Laurent) which also contains sandalwood. (See Chapter Ten for more.)

• Applications: topically, orally.

• Myrrh oil is found in:
7th Heaven Kit (Humility™, White Angelica™), Exodus II™, 3 Wise Men™, Abundance™, Hope™

Available from: Care Publications, RR 4, Box 646, Marble Hill, MO 63764
(573) 238-4846 • <care@clas.net> • Price: $19.95 + 6 s&h

9. MYRTLE
Myrtus communis   **Family: Murtaceae**

• Scriptures: Nehemiah 8:15; **Esther 2:7** (a Hebrew name for Esther was Hadassah, meaning Myrtle.) Isaiah 41:19; 55:13; Zechariah 1:7-11

• Source: From the leaves of the tree

• Chemistry: Monoterpenes: alpha Pinene, Monoterpene alcohols; Terpene oxides: Cineole; Sesquiterpenes; Ketones; Terpene esters

• Ancient Uses: Religious ceremony, purification from ritual uncleanliness

• Modern uses: Thyroid and general hormone balancer, soothing to respiratory system, decongestant, sinus infections, tuberculosis, colds, flu, coughs, bronchitis, asthma, skin conditions: acne, psoriasis, blemishes, bruises

• Applications: Inhaling, rubbing on chest, diffusing, suitable for children

• Myrtle oil is found in:
7th Heaven Kit (Inspiration™), Endoflex™, Purification™, R.C.™

"After this the Lord appointed seventy others and sent them on ahead of him in pairs to every town and place where he himself intended to go. He said to them . . . heal the sick that are therein and say to them 'The Kingdom of God has come near to you'." Luke 10:1-2, 9

---

10. ONYCHA
Styrax benzoin   Family: Styracaceae

• Scriptures: Exodus 30:34 (also in Talmud and Old Testament Apocrypha: Sirach 24:15)

• Source: From resin of tree.

• Chemistry: Phenolic Aldehydes: Benzoic aldehyde and Vanillin; Esters; Phenolic Acids: Benzoic and Cinnamic; Diterpenes; Triterpenes. Di- and Tri-terpenes are not commonly found in essential oils except in trace quantities. They are heavier than Mono- and Sesquiterpenes. This makes onycha the most viscous of all the oils. The heavier terpenes also give color to plants, fruits and flowers and give a golden color to Onycha. Vanillin aldehyde gives onycha its characteristic aroma. Also called: "Benzoin," "Friar's Balsam," and "Java Frankincense."

• Ancient Uses: Perfume, blended in holy anointing oils, comforting, soothing, uplifting, an ointment to heal skin wounds. Used as a fixative.

• Modern Uses: Stimulates renal output, used for colic, flatulence, constipation, and may help control blood sugar levels. Inhaled for sinusitis, bronchitis, colds, coughs, and sore throats. Soothing, used for dermatitis and skin wounds. Relieves stress when used in massage.

• Applications: Inhaled, use in massage, applied topically, in wound dressings.

• Available only in "Oils of Ancient Scriptures Kit."

---

11. ROSE OF SHARON/CISTUS/ROCK ROSE
Cistus ladanifer   Family: Cistaceae

• Scriptures: Song of Solomon 2:1 (The rose mentioned in Isaiah 35:1 is another species. See Chapter Eight.) See Genesis 37:25 and 43:11 where Myrrh is mentioned in English, but the Hebrew word in this passage is ladanum, which is actually Rock Rose or Rose of Sharon.

• Source: From Branches

• Chemistry: Monoterpenes: alpha Pinene, Camphene; Aldehydes; Ketones.

• Ancient Uses: Elevating moods, perfume

• Modern Uses: Antiseptic, immune enhancing, neurotonic, aids in normal cell regeneration, calming to nerves. Monoterpenes reprogram cellular memory thus promoting permanent healings. Notice that the monoterpene alpha Pinene is also found in Myrtle, Galbanum, Frankincense, Cypress, and Spikenard and may be the principal component responsible for the reprogramming function in all of these oils.

• Applications: Diffuse or use topically with massage oil.

• Rose of Sharon is available under the name of "Cistus oil" and is an ingredient in Immupower™

"Is any sick among you? Let him call for the elders of the church; and let them pray over him, anointing him with oil in the name of the Lord." James 5:14

---

12. SPIKENARD
Nardostachys jatamansi
Family: Valerianaceae

• Scriptures: Song of Solomon 1:12; 4:13, 14
Matthew 26:6-7; Luke 7:36-38; Mark 14:3
John 12:1-3

• Source: From plant roots

• Chemistry: Sesquiterpenes 93%—the third
highest in sesquiterpenes of all known oils (Only
Cedarwood 98% and Vetiver 97% have more,
while Sandalwood has 90%); Esters: Bornyl
acetate and Isobornyl valerianate; Phenols; Alpha
Pinene (also contained in Cistus, Cypress,
Frankincense, Galbanum and Myrtle.)

• Ancient Uses: Perfumes, medicines, skin tonic,
incense, mood enhancer, reduces anxiety. One of
the last oils to be received by Jesus before being
arrested and going to the cross, perhaps to help
prepare him for his ordeal. Heals scar tissue.

• Modern Uses: Allergies, migraine, nausea, cardiovascular support, tachycardia, relaxing,
soothing, emotionally calming. Mood elevating.

• Application: Applied to abdomen, on location,
inhaled, on feet, on head.

• Spikenard is found in:
7th Heaven Kit (Humility™), Exodus II™

"And they anointed with oil many that were sick, and
healed them." Mark 6:13

Available from: Care Publications, RR 4, Box 646, Marble Hill, MO 63764
(573) 238-4846 • <care@clas.net> • Price: $19.95 + 6 s&h

Bibliography

Books that we recommend as good sources of reliable information on aromatherapy, biochemistry, and the healing use of essential oils are noted with asterisks and their titles are given in boldfaced type.

Achtemeier, Paul, editor. (1985) *Harper's Bible Dictionary.* Society of *Bible* Literature, Harper Collins, New York. 1178 pp.

Anderson, A.W. (1956) *Plants of the Bible.* Crosby Lockwood & Son Ltd., London, England. 72 pp.

Archeological Institute of America. (1967) *Archeological Discoveries in the Holy Land.* Bonanza Books, New York. 219 pp.

Asala, Joanne (2002) *Foods from the Bible*, American Mecia, Boca Raton, FL. 96 pp.

National Council of Churches in Christ. (1957) T*he Old Testament Apocrypha, Revised Standard Version.* Thomas Nelson Publishers, New York. 250 pp.

Auerbach, Leo, translator. (1944) T*he Babylonian Talmud.* Philosophical Library, New York. 286 pp.

Buttrick, George. (1962) *The Interpreter's Dictionary of the Bible,* 4 vols. Abingdon Press, Nashville, TN. 3500 pp.

Carper, Jean. (1988) *The Food Pharmacy.* Bantam Books, New York. 256 pp.

Centre Informatique et *Bible.* (1983) *Concordance to the Apocrypha/Deuterocanonical Books.* Forward by Bruce M. Metzger, Wm. Eerdmans Publishing Co. Grand Rapids, MI. 504 pp.

Charlesworth, James H. editor. (1983) *The Old Testament Pseudepigrapha*, vol. s, doubleday 7 Co., Garden city, NY. 992 pp.

Dirsin, Denise, editor. (1996) *What Life was Like on the Banks of the Nile: Egypt (3050-30 B.C.),*Time-Life Books, Richmond, VA. 192 pp.

Dobilis, Inge, project editor. (1986) *The Magic and Medicine of Plants*, Readers Digest Assoc., Pleasantville, NY. 461 pp.

* Friedmann, Terry Shepherd. (2002) *The Man Who Walked With Jesus, Tales from the Sixth Disciple (Matthew).*Harvest Publishing, Denver, Colorado. 289 pp.

* Higley, Connie & Alan. (2003) *Reference Guide for Essential Oils.* 7th edition, Abundant Health Publications, Orem, UT. 547 pp.

Hitter, Greg (2001) History and Practice of Smudging. Personal communication via email, 12-17-01.

Holmes, Peter (1995) *Frankincense: The Rainbow Bridge.* Article from Greg Hitter. 6 pp.

Laymon, Charles M., editor. (1971) *Interpreter's One-Volume Commentary on the Bible and Apocrypha.* Abingdon Press, Nashville, TN 1385 pp.

Lynn, Jim. (2000) *Power for Healing Workshop Syllabus.* Power for Healing Workshop, Rockford, IL. 50 pp.

* Lynn, Jim. (2002) *The Miracle of Healing in Your Church Today.* Lynn Publications, Rockford, IL. 300 pp.

McMahon, Christopher. (2002) *Adventure with Frankincense.* Aromatherapy Journal, Vol. 12, No. 1, pp. 17-20

* Manwaring, Brian, editor. (2004) *Essential Oils Desk Reference*, 3rd edition. Essential Science Publishing, Orem, UT. 511 pp.

May, Herbert and Metzger, Bruce, editors. (1973) *The New Oxford Annotated Bible with the Apocrypha (RSV),* Oxford University press, NY. 298 pp.

McBride, Janet. (2001) *Scriptural Essence: Secrets of the Cohanim.* Essential Opportunities, Phoenix, AZ. 35 pp.

McDougall, John A. (1990) *The McDougal Program,* Penguin Books, NY. 433 pp.

* Mein, Carolyn L. (1999) *Releasing Emotional Patterns with Essential Oils*, 3rd edition, VisionWare Press, Rancho Sante Fe, CA. 107 pp.

Mendelsohn, Robert S. (1979) *Confessions of a Medical Heretic,* Contemporary Books, Chicago, 191 pp.

* Penoel, Daniel and Rose-Marie. (1998) *Natural Home Health Care Using Essential Oils.* (trans., rev. & enlarged from, *Pratique Aromatique Familiale,* 1992, Brian Manwaring, editor, Essential Science Publishing, Orem, UT. 236 pp.

Pert, Candace. (1999) **Molecules of Emotion**, Touchstone Books, New York. 368 pp.

* Price, Shirley and Len. (1999) *Aromatherapy for Health Professionals,* second ed. Churchill Livingston, New York. 391 pp.

Robbers, James, Speedie, Marilyn, and Tyler, Varroe. (1996) *Pharmacognosy and Pharmacobiotechnology.* Williams & Wilkins, Baltimore, MD. 337 pp.

Rose, Jeanne. (1999) 375 *Essential Oils and Hydrosols.* Frog, Ltd., Berkeley, CA. 251 pp.

Rutgers Media. (2001) *Myrrh, Fragrant Resin with Ancient Heritage,* May Bear Anti-Cancer Agents. Rutgers Univ., http://ur.rutgers.edu/medrel/ Dec. 6, 2 pp.

* Schnaubelt, Kurt. (1999) *Medical Aromatherapy.* Frog Ltd., Berkeley, CA. 296 pp.

Scholem, Gershom G. (1965) *Jewish Gnosticism, Merkabah Mysticism and Talmudic Tradition,* Jewish Theological Seminary of America, NY. 136 pp.

Shaw, Jerry .(2001) *The Healing Power of Olive Oil.* American Media, Inc., Boca Raton, FL. 63 pp.

Shutes, Jade. (2001) *What's Natural About Natural?* Aromatherapy Journal, Vol. 11, No. 2, Autumn issue. p. 24

* Smith, Linda. (2003) *Healing Oils, Healing Hands*. HTSM Press, Arvada, Colorado. 264 pp.

Steinsaltz, Adin. (1976) *The Essential Talmud.* Bantam Books, New York. 296 pp.

Stewart, David. (1977) *The Limits of Science in Medicine.* Chapter in the book, "21st Century Obstetrics," Vol. 2, Napsac Reproductions, Marble Hill, MO. pp. 281-310

Stewart, David. (1997) *Five Standards for Safe Childbear-ing,* revised fourth edition, Napsac Reproductions, Marble Hill, MO. 536 pp.

Stewart, David. (2001) *Longevity is a Bowl of Berries and a Drop of Clove.* Raindrop Messenger, Center for Aroma-therapy Research and Education, Marble Hill, MO. September issue. pp. 6-10.

• Stewart, David. (2003) *A Statistical Validation of Raindrop Technique.* Care Publications, Marble Hill, MO. 63 pp.

Stewart, David. (2004) *The Chemistry of Essential Oils Made Simple*. Care Publications, Marble Hill, Missouri. 425 pp.

Strong, James. *Strong's Exhaustive Concordance of the Bible,* Hendrickson Publishers, Peabody, Massachusetts. 1440 pp.

Tisserand, Robert.(1977) *The Art of Aromatherapy.* Healing Arts Press, Rochester, VT. 321 pp.

Tompkins, Peter, and Bird, Christopher. (1972) *The Secret Life of Plants.* Harper & Row, New York. 402 pp.

Truman, Karol K. (1995) *Feelings Buried Alive Never Die,* revised edition, Olympus Distributing, Las Vegas, NV. 298 pp.

* Valnet, Jean. (1982) *The Practice of Aromatherapy*. R. Tisserand, editor. Healing Arts Press, Rochester, VT. 279 pp.

Watt, Martin, & Sellar, Wanda. (1996) *Frankincense and Myrrh*. C.W. Daniel Co. Ltd., Essex, England.112 pp.

Weil, Andrew. (1995) *Spontaneous Healing*. Alfred Knopf Publisher, New York. 186 pp.

Wright, Henry. (2000) *A More Excellent Way: The Spiritual Roots of Disease*, fifth edition, Pleasant Valley Church, Molena, GA. 316 pp.

* Young, D. Gary. (1996) *Aromatherapy: The Essential Beginning,* second ed. Essential Science Publishing, Orem, UT. 174 pp.

* Young, D. Gary. (1999) *Introduction to Essential Oils,* sixth edition, Essential Oils, Inc., Payson, UT. 117 pp.

Young, D. Gary. (1999) *Level I Distributor Training Materials.* Essential Oils, Inc., Payson, UT. 70 pp

Young, D. Gary. (1999) *Level II Distributor Training Materials.* Essential Oils, Inc., Payson, UT. 90 pp

Young, D. Gary. (2000) *Twelve Oils of Ancient Scripture.* (Brochure) Essential Oils, Inc., Payson, UT. 6 pp.

Young, D. Gary. (2001) *Oils of Scripture.* (Audio Tape) Essential Oils, Inc., Payson, UT. 60 min.

* Young, D. Gary. (2003) *Essential Oils Integrative Medical Guide*. Essential Science Publishing, Essential Science Publishing, Orem, UT. 610 pp.

Young, Robert. (1982) *Young's Analytical Concordance to the Bible.* Thomas Nelson Publishers, New York. 1202 pp.

Young Life Research Clinic. (2001) *Why Essential Fatty Acids are Essential for Health.* Natural Medicine Alert, Institute of Natural Medicine, Springville, UT. January. pp. 9-15

Young Life Research Clinic. (2001) *Fruits that Prevent Cancer and Premature Aging.* Institute of Natural Medicine, Springville, UT. Feb/Mar issue. pp. 1-8

Zohary, Michael. (1962) *Plant Life of Palestine.* Ronald Press, New York. 262 pp.

Principal *Bibles* Consulted and Abbreviations Used:
   Authorized King James Version (KJV),
   New Revised Standard Version (NRSV)

Other *Bibles* Consulted:
   New International Version (NIV).
   New King James Version (NKJV),
   Revised Standard Version (RSV),
   *King James Easy-Reading Study *Bible* (KJERS)

*The KJERS edition of the *Bible* is the KJV with all of the Elizabethan English (thee, thine, blesseth, etc.) changed into Modern English (you, yours, blessed, etc.) and where the archaic words of the KJV are retained but are defined in modern language alongside the verses where they occur. (cf. Proverbs 17:20 where "froward," an archaic term, is clarified in the KJERS by the modern words, "crooked or deceitful." The KJERS also contains many articles of history, definition, and explanation, along with many cross-references, that are very helpful to students of the *Bible*. It was published in 2002 by G.E.M. Publishing, Goodyear, Arizona.

Index

About the Author

D r. David Stewart studied theology, philosophy, and English literature at Central Methodist College in Fayette, Missouri (1955–58) and studied chemistry, biology, and social sciences at Central Missouri State University in Warrensburg (1962–63). He also studied commercial photography at Los Angeles Trade Technical College (1959-60). He completed a BS degree in Mathematics and Physics at Missouri School of Mines and Metallurgy in 1965 and was salutatorian of his graduating class. His MS and PhD degrees are in geophysics (theoretical seismology) and were earned from the University of Missouri at Rolla in 1969 and 1971 respectively.

He spent a semester in medical school at the University of North Carolina (1973) and has been a Certified Childbirth Educator (CCE) with the American Academy of Husband-Coached Childbirth (AAHCC) since 1975. He has spent some 300 hours in training with Dr. Gary Young (ND)— internationally recognized authority on aromatherapy, essential oil production, and the originator of raindrop technique.

Dr. Stewart is also a Registered Aromatherapist (RA) with the Aromatherapy Registration Council (ARC), which is endorsed by the National Association of Holistic Aromatherapists (NAHA), of which he is a professional member.

He has held positions as a hydraulic engineer and hydrologist with the U.S. Geological Survey in Southern California (1965-67). He was a professor on the faculty of the University of North Carolina, Chapel Hill (1971–1978) where he was director of the MacCarthy Geophysics Laboratory. He also held a professorship at Southeast Missouri State University, Cape Girardeau (1988–1993) where he was founder and director of the Center for Earthquake Studies. He was a part-time United Methodist Pastor (1993–94, 1997–99) in rural Missouri. He has been the Executive Director of the InterNational Association of Parents and Professionals for Safe Alternatives in Childbirth (NAPSAC International) since its founding in 1975.

For most of his professional career he has been self-employed as an author and lecturer, mainly in the area of alternative health care. He has served on advisory committees to the American Public Health Association (APHA) and the American College of Nurse-Midwives (ACNM). He has testified as an expert on health matters before state legislative committees, U.S. congressional committees, medical licensing boards, and courts of law throughout the U.S. and Canada.

He has authored or co-authored over 200 published works, including sixteen books. Two of his books won the "Books of the Year" Award from the *American Journal of Nursing.* One of his flyers on breastfeeding (published by La Leche League International, LLLI) sold over two million copies in ten languages.

As a lecturer, he has spoken throughout the U.S. and Canada and given international presentations in Lima, Peru, on behalf of the Pan American Health Organization (PAHO) and in Bogota, Colombia, on behalf of the United Nations Disaster Relief Organization (UNDRO). He has been quoted in newspapers and magazines throughout the U.S. and has made numerous radio interviews. He has appeared on television in 44 countries.

As a Registered Aromatherapist and Executive Director for the Center for Aromatherapy Research and Education (CARE), he conducts research and training seminars leading to status as a Certified CARE Instructor (CCI) throughout North America. His courses include: Healing Oils of the *Bible*, Raindrop Technique, Applied Vitaflex, Aromachemistry, and Emotional Release with Essential Oils. If you would like to learn more about CARE's programs, attend one of Dr. Stewart's seminars, or if you would like to arrange for Dr. Stewart to do a program in your area, contact CARE and express your interest: (See pp. 324-325 of this book.)

CARE, RR 4, Box 646, Marble Hill, MO 63764
(573) 238-4846 • care@clas.net
• www.RaindropTraining.com •

Dr. Stewart lives on a farm in Southeast Missouri with his wife, Lee. They have been married since September 1962 and have five children. They also have eight grandchildren. They attend the Marble Hill United Methodist Church where Lee is church treasurer, plays the piano, and directs the choir and where David sings tenor, plays the organ, and teaches Sunday School from time to time.

"The more I pour over your book, *Healing Oils of the Bible*, the more I see what an awesome piece of work it is. You have assembled so many elements, kept it simple, and focused on the heart of the message. Solid reasoning throughout."

Kathy Spohn, CCI
Wyoming, Michigan

"Dr. Stewart has done his homework. His delivery of hundreds of *Bible* references to essential oils, combined with their uses, is clear, concise, enjoyable, and fun. He has a rare gift for integrating, synthesizing, and applying vast amounts of information. A must read for anyone interested in the Biblical bases of healing with oils."

John Maeder and Marilee Tolen, RN, HNC
Atco, New Jersey

"I have just received my first 20 copies of *Healing Oils of the Bible*. WOW! Dr. Stewart has done a fantastic job of getting tons of information into one great resource for anyone using oils. The appendices are fantastic. So rich, so thorough. I got so excited, I had to get out my scriptural oils and start anointing myself. I kept my blend of oils from Exodus in my pocket the whole time I read the book. Dr. Stewart outlines a great *Bible* Oils program at the end that you can do in your community. Anyone could do the program with this helpful text. Even me. I learned so much! What a great book!"

Jacquelyn Close, CCI, RA, Director
Center for Conscious Healing
Jackson, Missouri

"My first copy of *Healing Oils of the Bible* arrived while I was at ministerial school. After classes ended for the term, I took one week to vegetate and what did I do but to read and reread this fabulous book. My friends who were ordained during this session have now all received this book as a gift from me. In fact, this book is one of the main gifts I give away to everyone now. I quote from it constantly."

Rev. Terrie Woznicki
Cicero, Illinois